BIORHYTHM
for Health Design

by Kichinosuke Tatai, M.D., M.P.H.

Japan Publications, Inc.

© in Japan 1977 *by* Kichinosuke Tatai

Published by
JAPAN PUBLICATIONS, INC., Tokyo, Japan

Distributed by
JAPAN PUBLICATIONS TRADING COMPANY
200 Clearbrook Road, Elmsford, N. Y. 10523, U.S.A.
1174 Howard Street, San Francisco, Calif. 94103, U.S.A.
P.O. Box. 5030 Tokyo International, Tokyo 101–31, Japan

First edition: March, 1977

ISBN 0–87040–393–1
LCCC No. 76–029337

Printed in Japan by Kyodo Printing Co., Ltd.

Preface

Both time and life are currents in themselves. Biology posits chronology; that is, chronology is the basic system of all biology. When I was in high school, I was deeply impressed by Thomas Mann's *Der Zauberberg* and especially by the first part of Chapter VI, in which the hero, Hans Kastorp, reflects on the meaning of time. He says that time is the greatest mystery. It is never substantial, but always almighty. Present is no more past. Here is no more there. Without doubt, time is cyclic. The past is always repeated in the present. He ponders the means by which the finite existence is harmonized in the universe. The thoughts expressed in this passage influenced my decision to study psychology and physiology and ultimately led me to the study of timing in the living system. My doctoral thesis, presented to the Medical Faculty of Tokyo University in 1947, was on the subject "Human Ability to Adapt to Seasonal Changes." Since the time of that thesis, I have devoted myself to research in human stress, circadian rhythms, and microcirculatory rhythms.

In the initial stage of my life as a research scientist, shortly after my graduation from Tokyo University, I came into contact with Wilhelm Fliess's biorhythm theory. In the section entitled "*Periodentheorie*" in Willy Hellpach's *Geopsyche*, I read that, in his elaborate clinical experiments at the beginning of this century, Fliess had discovered certain cycles that were twenty-three days long for males and twenty-eight days long for females.

My interest was revived in this subject in the early 1960's, when I was eagerly searching for means to reduce the increasing number of traffic accidents occurring in Japan. At that time, I investigated the autogenic training system created in the 1930's by Johannes Heinrich Schultz. His system is related to psychosomatic medicine and was developed under the influence of Zen, Buddhism, and Yoga. As a member of the Japanese Society of Psychosomatic Medicine and as the Japanese representative to the International Association for Suicide Prevention, first of all, I felt that this system would be helpful in my campaign against traffic accidents.

Human beings are accustomed to think in terms of numerical segmentations. For instance, in the West, the seven-day cycle is deep-rooted and ancient. In the Orient, on the other hand, the most ancient cycle is six days. During that period, there is customarily one highly auspicious day, a time when people plan weddings and other ceremonies. There is also one very ill-omened day when the people avoid all ceremonies. Of course, these customs are entirely superstitious; but they have had one practical social influence: people who provide services for various ceremonies are busy on auspicious days and idle on unlucky days.

The cycles dealt with in this book—physical, sensitivity, and intellectual cycles of the biorhythm, or PSI theory—are not matters of superstition. Scientific work in Germany, the United States, the United Kingdom, Japan, and other nations is currently under way to provide further detailed information about their natures. I hope that the readers of this book will find it interesting. But more important, I hope the book will convince more people of the importance of biorhythm and the contributions it can make to life and happiness.

I should like to say at this point that I do not like the word *biorhythm* in connection with the PSI theory because it is too broad in application and too vague for strict scientific use. I am inclined to propose such words as *neo-Fliessian* or *triperiodic human potentiality*. Terms of this kind do not suggest fortune-telling, but indicate a conscious biofeedback with sensible motivations. But, since biorhythm is currently popular, I have used it here as suitable to an introductory text of this kind.

In concluding these remarks, I should like to offer my warmest thanks to Iwao Yoshizaki, president of the Japan Publications, Inc.; to Miss Yotsuko Watanabe, editoress; and to Richard L. Gage, who translated the text into English.

March, 1977

KITCHINOSUKE TATAI

Contents

Part 1

Basic
Considerations

Life Rhythms

Lower unicellular organisms live in rhythms of activity and repose. In higher organisms, to these fundamental rhythms are added the rhythmical alteration of generations in reproductive and somatic cells. All of this is governed by the flow of life. If this flow is disturbed, such potentially fatal illness as cancer can easily develop. In the following pages, I shall concentrate on the importance of data related to biorhythm, the biological clock that governs activity and repose.

In biological terms, the eternal flow of life on earth is best seen in the reproductive cells. At maturity, the male produces sperm cells and the female ova. When an ovum is fertilized by a sperm cell, cellular division begins and advances until the embryo is formed. At birth, the developed embryo becomes the infant, which grows until adolescence and then matures to become capable of producing further reproductive cells. Thereafter, the human being grows through adulthood to old age and ultimately death. This is the process that life-insurance companies refer to as the life cycle.

But, in this case *cycle* is not an accurate term, because human beings, like all other living organisms, die once and for all. No second opportunity for life is granted. No human life can be repeated. Nor is a human life merely a long, unbroken current, for each part of it, each instant in it, is unique and cannot be relived. Though one morning or one evening may seem very much like another, in the individual life, there can be no duplication. We travel a one-way street, for the old man can never again become an infant.

The story is different with reproductive cells. Although they rarely appear in the world of phenomena, reproductive cells rejuvenate. A fertilized ovum is, at the first instant, unicellular; but cell division begins at once. Most of the new cells produced by division are somatic; but some of them become reproductive cells, which are activated when the individual reaches the age of sexual maturity. It is biologically true that, as the old Japanese song says, the father is only the shell of the son. In other words, reproductive cells operate in a constantly recurring and eternal cycle made up of long periods of immaturity and brief periods of maturity. In comparison with this everlasting flow, the individual life is only a shell that comes into this world for a period of roughly seventy years.

Today warfare threatens life all over the globe, and man's heedless actions have drastically polluted the natural environment. As part of a drive to do something to halt both of these destructive trends, much attention is currently being devoted to a study of the nature of life. As of yet, however, no one has performed the kind of research on the subject that was done by Aleksandr Ivanovich Oparin (born in 1894). According to this great Soviet biochemist, life first came into being three billion years ago, in the confusion of roaring skies and trembling earth when lightning flashed through the air over the still-fluid surface of the newly formed world. In the succeeding three billion years, life silently evolved. Probably in those distant times, the amoeba that was someday to develop into man possessed a higher degree of adaptability than its other amoeba counterparts. From the first amino acids making up nuclear substance, life advanced to the amoeba, the prototypical organism. Then, with the division of the surface of the earth into seas and land masses, organisms suited to aquatic and land environments evolved. At last man came into being. But, in comparison with the total history of life on earth, his duration has been only a brief two hundred thousand years.

The true point of origin of the rhythm of life is to be found in the alternation of generations seen in the recurrent phases of sexual maturity and immaturity. Human beings are often so engrossed in the affairs of the world that they tend to interpret the significance of life in terms of their own activities, their happiness and sorrow, their loves and hates, their altruism and their cruelty. But this approach is groundless because the true origin of life is found in the reproductive cells. The mental and physical activities of human beings are no more than the hull produced by life. The relation between the two is similar to that between the snail and its shell. To interpret actions and phenomena as humanity is to lose sight of the basic issue. Human beings reach maturity and must fade, as flowers that have reached full bloom, must fall. But man leaves his reproductive cells in the form of the next generation.

All geophysicists agree that, within the rhythmical alteration of generations, the earth rotates on its axis once every twenty-four hours. Physiologists are unanimous in recognizing the power of the daily rhythm of light and dark resulting from these rotations to stimulate evolution in life. Some creatures, like cockroaches and rats, because they are affected by periods of light and dark in ways that differ from those experienced by man, become nocturnal in habits. Other animals, reacting like man, are directly stimulated by the sunlight to evolve as diurnal creatures.

Upsetting the long-established day-and-night, twenty-four-hour rhythm of the earth invariably produces some kind of abnormality in the living organism. Dr. W. Yeffle, who works at the German Schelling Pharmaceutical Laboratory, reports that continued exposure to light stimulates the generation of breast cancer in female rats. Continued light produces cancer in rats in fifty days earlier on an average. Transferred into terms of human life, this means that, in a human being, the illness would occur four years earlier than it might be expected ordinarily and that death would occur three years earlier.

Research by the English zoologist Dr. Janet E. Harker has proved that reversal of the day-and-night rhythm produces cancer in the intestines of the cockroach, one of the most representative nocturnal creatures. She raised one group of cockroaches under artificially controlled conditions of light at night and dark in the day until the insects were completely accustomed to this rhythm. Then she removed nerve ganglia from below the esophagus of each of the cockroaches and transplanted them into cockroaches that had been raised under normal conditions of light by day and dark by night. In four days after the transplantation, all of the cockroaches that were kept on the normal rhythm had developed cancer. Transplantation of ganglia from cockroaches raised under the normal rhythm to others raised under the same rhythm did not produce cancer. Obviously, the joint existence in the body of two dark-light rhythms caused the illness. Without doubt, the hormone secreted at the command of the ganglia for the control of day and night activities intervened in this pathological change.

It has been shown that alterations in the day-night rhythm of rats upset hormone control and, in this way, detonate pathological change. Professor Franz Halberg of the University of Minnesota showed that artificially accelerating the earth's twenty-four-hour rotational pattern by eight hours causes rats to experience stress and disturbs thier hormone secretions.

For three billion years, the day-and-night rhythm of the earth has controlled all living things from the smallest unicellular organisms to man. Like the workings of a great clock, the rhythm has established what is called biorhythm. Information about ways to stay in harmony with biorhythm can be a great advantage in daily life.

Discussion of these rules brings us to the nervous and endocrine systems, the two major systems for controlling mental and physical well-being. I have been studying this subject for thirty years; and, in the following text, I should like to put to use the information I have gained as a consequence of this study in the hope that it will be of use to you in daily life.

The graph below shows alterations in the diameter of the pupil of the eye during the course of twenty-four hours as measured by Dr. Gerd Döring of Munich University. Using a mirror and a specially designed device, Dr. Döring measured the pupil eight times a day at intervals of three hours. In the graph, the small circular marks represent mean values; the vertical rods at the circles indicate individual differentials. As can easily be seen, the pupil is open widest at eight in the morning and tends to contract after eight in the evening.

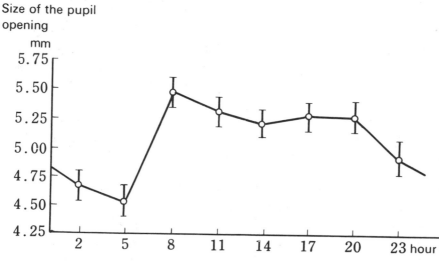

Changes in the diameter of the pupil of the eye in a twenty-four-hour period

The opening and narrowing of the pupil is performed by smooth muscles, which are not subject to voluntary control. When a person is tense, the sympathetic nerves and stimulative hormones, like adrenalin, go to work to contract the smooth muscles controlling the opening of the pupil. As the muscles contract, the opening of the pupil expands. In contrast, at night when a person becomes sleepy, the smooth muscles relax; and the opening of the pupil becomes smaller. But the automatic actions of the hormones and the nerves can make it possible to work well as long as the mind and the body are intent on the task at hand.

Obviously there are individual differences in capabilities. But, for the person to work to the best of his abilities, his condition must be right. Though some people are not aware of it, morning is usually the time at which most efficient and productive work is performed. This is proof that, over the ages, man has evolved as a diurnal creature.

An English scholar has clearly proved that there is a difference between morning and evening reading efficiency. If it takes a person ten seconds to read a line at eight in the morning, at four in the afternoon, it will take the same person fourteen seconds to read the same line. In other words, efficiency will have dropped by 40 percent.

Disruptions in biorhythm can cause malfunctioning in plants and can generate cancers in rats and cockroaches. Whether such irregularity can cause pathological changes in man has not been proved. But, especially since the end of World War II, a condition called night-work sickness (*Nachtarbeiterkrankheit*), brought on by disturbance of living rhythms has aroused great interest. Frequent reports of heart, stomach, intestinal, and liver ailments among shift workers in Germany prompted Japanese scholars to devote attention to this condition. It was found that people who work nights for long periods tend to lose appetite; and, in the case of people with highly sensitive autonomic nerves, ulcers of the stomach and duodenum often result. German statistics state that cases of stomach ulcer are eight times more frequent in people who work a shift system than in day workers and that ordinary stomach complaints are four times more frequent. Heart sicknesses may arise in people who work at night because this is the time at which the energy supplied by the joint actions of the nervous and endocrine systems tends to decrease. Though systolic (maximum) pressure and pulse decrease, diastolic (minimum) pressure does not decrease; this lowers the efficiency of the blood circulation and brings on attacks like angina pectoris. The German scientist Dr. Alexander Pierach claims that such attacks are twice as frequent among night workers as among day workers.

Hormones that influence the upset of life rhythms include, in addition to the stimulative adrenalin and the adrenal cortex hormones, thyroxine, produced by the thyroid gland. Because of their role in making possible the production of a fairly large infant in a ten-month gestation period, the hormones and alterations in their secretion are of greater significance in the female than in the male. During World War II, women employed in communications organizations of the German defense forces followed a schedule in which they worked the same shift for three days and then changed. Within four or five weeks of this schedule, many of the women were stricken with Basedow's (or Graves's) disease and suffered from sleeplessness, headaches, and irritability.

From my standpoint as a specialist in health designs, damaging health and causing sickness by upsetting the biorhythm governing the twenty-four hours of all human days is deeply related to daily living capabilities. I place a rational living plan based on the application of biorhythm at the top of the list in what I call "The Economics of Health." For instance, even though you may feel sluggish, sleepy, or tired, the stimulative hormones and the autonomic nervous system do not fall down on their job of keeping you active and lively in the early morning. If you have a piece of important or creative work that must be accomplished, take advantage of the morning phase to do it. In the afternoon, if the sluggishness persists, do only light, simple work. If you feel very tired, do not hesitate to rest. Even though it may not yet be time to quit, if you have used your morning energy to the full, stopping a little early will have no detrimental effect on your output.

It is important to bear in mind the effect of what I am saying on people other than ordinary salaried workers. It applies equally to leaders of all kinds. I am convinced that holding important conferences on commercial or national matters in the afternoon can bring about disaster. The leaders who participate in these conferences are likely to fall victim to the so-called managerial sickness produced by the stresses under which they must live. People who attempt to accomplish as much as possible even at conferences that take place in the afternoon when everyone's efficiency is low often lie awake at night because of overactive hormones and nerves. Before they realize what is happening, they find their health impaired.

The way to use biorhythm to live an ordered life is to follow the instructions of the providence that has guided life on earth for three billion years. In a sense this is like being able to ride surf. The content of the providence is abundant. The biorhythm of which I have been speaking is easy for the ordinary person to understand. But it is also a field in which biologists and medical doctors have already conducted a complete course of research.

Monthly cycles of physiological change are known to most people as a consequence of the female menstrual cycle, controlled by sex-related hormone secretions. Dr. Karl Birzele of Graz University has made detailed studies by means of Rorschach tests and other methods on the twenty-seven-day activity cycle influenced by the cyclical behavior of sun spots.

But in this book I intend to deal with biorhythm in the narrow sense of the PSI (physical, sensitivity, and intellctual cycles) theory. At present some scholars doubt the validity of this theory or activily oppose it with theories of their own. It has been over ten years since I first conducted social experiments with the PSI theory in Japan. As a result of my experiments, I believe the hypothesis on which the theory rests has been proved. In the following chapters, I shall discuss biorhythm from the fundamental and the applied standpoints and shall analyze it in connection with possible future investigation.

The Theory Begins with Dr. W. Fliess

The theory that is accurately known as the theory of physical, sensitivity, and intellectual cycles (PSI) is more commonly referred to as the theory of biorhythm. It was first discoverd by Dr. Wilhelm Fliess (1859–1928), who was a specialist in ear and throat illness at the University of Berlin. A number of psychologists and engineering specialists followed up Fliess's work. The results of their efforts have been brought together under the name of the PSI theory. Some doctors and sports specialists in Europe used the theory to predict deterioration in patient's conditions and to try to improve performances of athletes. In 1939, after having examined the statistics on the subject, Dr. Hans Schwing suggested that biorhythm might be valuable in accident prevention.

Before beginning a discussion of the history of the development of biorhythm, I should like to make a few remarks about terminology. The word *biorhythm* is an abbreviation of *biological rhythms*. With the diffusion of the PSI theory developed by Dr. Wilhelm Fliess of the University of Berlin, *biorhythm* was assigned a narrower, more specialized meaning that people related to the field have come to approve. But, even used in connection with the narrow sense pertaining only to the PSI theory, the term is incorrect, for it ought to be biorhythmics (from the still more correct German *Biorhythmik*), or a study of biorhythm. The name *PSI* derives from the initials of the names of the three cycles with which it deals: physical cycle (twenty-three days); sensitivity, or emotional, cycle (twenty-eight days); and intellectual cycle (thirty-three days).

The word *rhythm* is used in the musical sense of regularity and repetition and always involves the time element. *Cycle* is used in a sense connected with regularity especially controlled by the time element. In biology, *cycle* is the more widely used word. But, since from the standpoint of phenomenology, this too can be understood to mean rhythm, it is impossible to make a strict distinction between the two terms.

Dr. Fliess, who first evolved the biorhythm theory, became the head of the Berlin Department of Sanitation and the chairman of the German Academy of Sciences. But he made the discovery of this theory while he was teaching nose-and-throat medicine at the University of Berlin. Examining the case histories of many of his patients, he seemed to discover regular cycles in the developments of their symptoms. To verify this, he called on a mathematician to analyze the statistics. In 1906, he discovered that this cycle of the development of sickness was twenty-three days for men and twenty-eight days for women. Dr. Fliess was on friendly terms with Dr. Sigmund Freud (1856–1939), who was then at the University of Vienna. Records are preserved of their discussions of cycles involving psychological elements.

Another professor of psychology at the University of Vienna, Dr. Herman Swoboda (1873–1963) discovered twenty-three-day and twenty-eight-day cycles in such things as pain and swelling caused by insect bites, fever in colds, and heart attacks. He insisted that there is a twenty-three-day cycle in male stamina and sexual potency and a twenty-eight-day cycle in relation to the characteristic emotional issues and sensitivities of women. Dr. Swoboda, who died in 1963 at the age of ninety, was granted honorary Viennese citizenship and was famous as the advocate of the unusual theory that racial mixtures result in genetic susceptibilities to cancer.

The work of these three men produced the idea that men and women are controlled by male (or physical) rhythms and by female (or emotional) rhythms. Since the science of endocrinology was not advanced at the time, some scholars objected to this theory; but today we realize that it was accurate and farsighted. Hormone measurements, which of course affect personality, show that men and women secrete both male and female hormones. In the male, there is usually, at most, twice the volume of male as of female hormones; whereas the female secretes five times as many female as male hormones.

Claude Bernard (1813–78), one of the fathers of modern experimental medicine, advanced the rule that a change in quantity brings about a change in quality. Modern science, symbolized by the computer, tends to regard all scientific changes as accumulations of volumes. But, at least in biology, including the study of human animals, the rule that a volume alteration is the cause of a qualitative alteration must not be overlooked. This rule is of fundamental importance to an understanding of biorhythm.

In 1928, Dr. Friedrich Teltscher, of the Engineering Department of the University of Innsbruck, used five thousand high-school and college students as subjects in experiments to prove the Fliess-Swoboda theory of physical and emotional cycles. In his report, he said that he had not only succeeded in proving the accuracy of the idea of these cycles, but had also uncovered a third, thirty-three-day cycle pertaining to the ability to remember and reason.

At about the same time, Dr. Lexford Hersey, of the University of Pennsylvania, conducted experiments on efficiency and accident prevention. He examined cyclical behavior in railway workers in relation to their emotional state, physical condition, and operational powers. In the numerous reports of his experiments, he both verified the twenty-three- and twenty-eight-day cycles and discovered a third, thirty-three-day cycle.

In the nineteen thirties, Dr. Alfred Judt, of Bremen University, devised a simple way of charting physical, emotional, and intellectual conditions from a person's date of birth. This method was used in sports training and by doctors in connection with the illnesses of patients. Then the Swiss engineer Hans Früh developed a calculating scale, based on the Judt chart. By means of this scale, great contributions were made to the study of accidents. Records have been preserved of the use of biorhythm in intensified training of German athletes before the prewar Berlin Olympics. Furthermore, soccer coaches have employed it in the past and continue to employ it today in training and selecting players. Doctors are able to use biorhythm to predict the time of death of cancer patients and in judging the best days on which to perform surgery. Employing a knowledge of the patient's biorhythm conditions, doctors have been able to prevent sudden, unpredictable, postsurgical hemorrhage or death. Dentists are able to reduce pain suffered by patients by avoiding days on which biorhythm indicates it would be unwise to extract teeth. Each of these topics will be treated separately in other parts of this book.

In 1939, Dr. Hans Schwing, working under the guidance of Dr. W. von Gonzenbach, of the Swiss National Institute of Technology, issued a thesis on biorhythm and its technological applications. His report dealt with seven hundred cases involving workers' accident insurance and with three hundred deaths in Zürich. He learned that, of the 700 accidents, 401 occurred on caution days; that is, days that biorhythm indicates demand great caution. Of the 300 deaths, 197 occurred on such days. European studies of biorhythm after World War II were conducted on the basis of the statistics gained from this report.

In 1954, the head instructor in the environmental sanitation department of the city of Hanover, Dr. Otto Tope, investigated accidents involving drivers of garbage trucks and watering trucks and discovered that 83 percent of them had occurred on days requiring caution from the biorhythm standpoint. Dr. Reinhold Bochow, of Humbolt University, in Berlin, studied 499 accidents involving people working with agricultural equipment and found that, on the average, many times more accidents occur on caution days than on ordinary days. None of the people he studied were lazy or careless. In spite of differences in experience, all of them were industrious and thoroughly familiar with their work. The accidents occurred because of unconsious oversights and slips. The report concluded that caution in connection with psychological elements could have prevented 62 percent of the accidents.

Before leaving this subject, I should like to relate an interesting episode that happened to me. In 1969, I was invited by the World Mental Health Association to take part in an international symposium on the subject of suicide. The meeting took place in Washington, D. C. As I was running up the seven or eight steps beside the entrance of my hotel in that city, the tip of my shoe hit the top step, and I fell. I thought little of the incident. But, on the following day, as I was once again running up the same steps, I stumbled and fell again. I walked down the steps and, one by one, measured the height of each riser. I learned that the topmost one was about two centimeters higher than the rest. It was not surprising that I stumbled: my feet, accustomed to risers of uniform height, suddenly encountered the obstacle of an extra two centimeters. Of course, discrepancies of this kind are carefully avoided in places where work safety is emphasized. I had not expected to find the hotel steps figuratively lying in ambush for me.

Unconsciously or not, the intelligent human animal always seeks to economize on daily activities. The many conditioned responses of daily living are proof of this. Such responses enable us to live more efficiently, but they can lead to the kind of unpleasant experience I had with the hotel steps. Many of the things we do become unconscious mannerisms, which are often indispensable from the viewpoint of activity economy. Biorhythm makes use of mannerisms to help foretell when mistakes and unpleasant occurrences will take place.

Progress in the Behavioral Science

The Western method for preventing accidents is based on the research in biorhythm influences by the Swiss Dr. Hans Schwing. It involves avoiding dangerous, or caution, days. Fifteen years ago, in Japan, I developed a new system making use of the autogenic training evolved by the German psychological medical expert Dr. Johannes H. Schultz. This new biorhythm system has had astounding success in preventing accidents. In many places of work, when the system was employed, accidents were reduced by as much as from one-third to three-fourths.

The introductory American article by Evan Juro, which appeared in translation in a popular Japanese magazine, in 1964, was probably the initial information on biorhythm offered by the Japanese mass-communications media. Shortly afterwards, when it became known that I was doing research in biorhythm, two or three people asked me to write articles on the subject. The National Land Defense Forces discussed the application of biorhythm systems as a result of these articles, but the discussions led to nothing definite.

In the spring of 1965, I wrote a book called *Seikatsu o Ayatsuru Shimpi na Rizumu* (The Mystic Rhythm Governing Daily Life). I was uncertain how much information on the PSI theory (biorhythm) to include in spite of many years of experiences with this theory. Many writers in the West lack elementary knowledge of biology and medicine. Consequently, their works on biorhythm contain doubtful material. Although I used some of their books as reference and as sources of some kinds of data, because of their largely unscientific content, I was unable to give them my total consent. Even in the article by Evan Juro there were exaggerations and deviations. In addition, thoroughly reliable scientific explanations of the subject were still incomplete and immature in some respects. In spite of the doubts aroused in me by the nature of this material, I decided to try to be impartial and to give a conservative explanation of the PSI theory because I considered it of great use to social welfare in general.

From the standpoint of practical science, the book stimulated many inquiries from readers. I suspect that this was because the Japanese people found something familiar in the idea of this rhythm. After all, the father of Western medicine, Hippocrates, placed great emphasis on ideas that can be said to resemble biological rhythms. More important from the Japanese standpoint, Chinese medicine, the core of all oriental medical thought, is filled with such ideas as the cycles of the seasons, the impossibility of escaping from the control of the cycles, and the importance of cyclic rhythm to health and long life.

In the West, study of biological rhythms as a science is comparatively new. It began in 1937 with the first conference of the International Society for Biological

Rhythms, held in Sweden. Similar meetings were held later in the Netherlands, Germany, Switzerland, and Italy. World War II interrupted the conferences, but they resumed with renewed vigor in the postwar period. Eight conferences have been held; and, in recent years, it has become customary to hold other special conferences and symposiums.

One of these was the Biological Rhythm Symposium sponsored by the New York Academy of Sciences in 1960. I was invited to attend that meeting. To stimulate expansion in the International Society for Biological Rhythms and the inclusion in its work of study of the entire range of the sciences, Dr. Solcow Tromp of the Netherlands now edits the quarterly *Journal of Interdisciplinary Cycle Research*. In support of this journal, international meetings are held every other summer. Between the time of its initial publication, in 1970, and 1976, six volumes of the quarterly were published. The editorial organization consists of a scientific fraternity of more than one hundred specialists from all over the world.

In the past twenty years, cosmological medicine has demanded special attention to the field of circadian rhythms (physiological rhythms associated with the twenty-four-hour cycle of the earth's rotation). These rhythms can be upset by many kinds of travel in which modern man engages, including of course such drastic cases as journeys to the moon and flights in supersonic military aircraft but extending to ordinary commercial travel by high-speed jet planes as well. The immense amounts of money poured into research in this field by the United States National Aeronautics and Space Agency (NASA) has inspired rapid progress in this and related areas. The astronauts in the Apollo project were trained, at Houston, Texas, to maintain a regular program of waking, sleeping, and eating. This pattern was the one they experienced in ordinary life on earth. Thanks to its application, Apollo astronauts were able to fulfill their missions and return safely to earth, though not without the fatal explosion of an oxygen tank and loss of lives in one instance.

When Richard Nixon made his important trip to Peking, in 1972, during the journey, he took three days of rest. This was to help him overcome upsets caused by disturbances in his biological rhythms resulting from time differences. It is likely that the days of rest contributed to the success of the conferences he held in China.

In terms of labor and money, biological-rhythms research is from ten to twelve times more costly than ordinary kinds of research. This is easy to understand when one takes into consideration the staggering figures involved in no more than surveying for biological-rhythms study. The passion for quick results that pervades much of the rest of society has invaded the world of research, and it is regrettable that little progress in biorhythm would be made if it were not for such special projects as cosmological medicine.

For more than thirty years after graduation from medical school, I devoted myself to the study of physiological adaptability of the human endocrine system and to stress reactions. My work in biorhythm arose as a consequence of the needs of this study. The subject of my doctoral thesis was adaptability to seasonal changes. I have studied activity rythms resulting from subtle alterations in the environment caused by circadian changes. Much of the work that I have presented to numerous international scholarly associations has centered on these subjects.

At a meeting in Europe more than a decade ago, I recalled the PSI theory and began to give it thought. At the time, many scholars looked askance at the theory. But it was interesting to me because I was attempting to understand the actual aspects of human stress reaction from the standpoint of mental health. In order to overcome stress and live in a healthy, happy way, one must face the stresscausing factor boldly and do away with it. It is no good running away in fear. Intuitively, I sensed that the PSI theory could be helpful in making such bold courage possible.

Although it has since become widely recognized, in those days, the autogenic training system of the specialist in psychologic medicine Dr. Johannes Heinrich Schultz, of the University of Berlin, was virtually unknown in Japan. In brief, this system strives to rebuild individual stress reactions on the basis of physiological sensations (In the United States this is now described by means of the term *biofeedback*). It seemed to me that, if the PSI theory could be applied to the same categories, stress would be easier to overcome.

My first impression was that the PSI theory was too mathematical. I later came to the conclusion that this was not the result of the intentions of Dr. Fliess. It was only that none of his successors had been men of biological and medical erudition. Further, I learned that, in the postwar period, commercial people without backgrounds in biology and medicine had willfully created something that completely ignored the original principles of biorhythm.

Following the lead of Dr. Fliess himself, I kept a record of my own caution days for a period of three years. Of course, in order to avoid autosuggestion, every month, I compared this with my PSI calendar. The result was an astoundingly high rate of accuracy about caution days. Since my youth, I have suffered from psychologically caused diarrhea. Occurrences of the sickness and my caution days coincided with an accuracy rate of more than 70 percent.

This personal experience probably ignited the spark for further research in biorhythm in Japan. I was able to talk about the significance of biorhythm with confidence because of my experience, which, through personal contacts with friends and through many other media, gradually reached a wide audience.

For more than ten years, I have been conducting accident-reduction plans with many commercial companies. These projects have been a kind of social experiment. By instituting a proper introduction of biorhythm, I have helped prove the effectiveness of autogenic training and have emphasized the human element in the system. These were my original intentions. The efforts of Edmund Husserl in philosophical phenomenology and the related *Biotakt* of Ludwig Klages have born fruit in that my work has added an element of morale and has proved the serviceability of behavioral science.

Unfortunately, however, though its serviceabilty has been proved, the contents of the PSI theory itself have not been analyzed sufficiently. As I have suggested already, much of the work on this subject up to the present has been absurd. More persevering research is needed to firm up the foundations of the PSI theory—which is still the target of scholarly criticism—and to improve the level of effectiveness of *Biotakt*.

For the Sake of the Future

Although the significance of the application to the behavioral science of biorhythm has been proved medically and in terms of various actual case histories, the nature of the purely biological rhythm itself remains unknown. In this section, I discuss some of the approaches to the problem. The most likely of the proposed explanations is the influence of the moon suggested by Dr. Hilmar Heckert and Dr. Curt Richter.

It must always be remembered that, as I pointed out in the section on its history, biorhythm was discovered by Dr. Fliess. It was he who, using case histories of a large number of patients, extracted twenty-three-and twenty-eight-day cycles in connection with physical and emotional conditions and in relation to such conditions as common colds, diarrhea, fever, heart attacks, apoplexy, hemorrhage, and childbirth. At present, however, we do not know why the physical cycle is twenty-three days, the emotional cycle twenty-eight days, and the intellectual cycle thirty-three days.

The twenty-eight-day cycle seems to be close to the average menstrual cycle. But closer examination shows that the average menstrual cycle tends to be twenty-nine and a half days; that is, closer to the lunar cycle itself. Furthermore, the twenty-eight-day biorhythm cycle occurs in girls who have not reached sexual maturity and in women who have passed menopause. The same cycle occurs in men. Though the range of fluctuation is less than in women, in highly emotional men, the cycle appears clearly. Observations of three-year health diaries of fifty college women showed that changes in menstrual cycle and emotional biorhythm are completely independent and unrelated. In short, in spite of numerous hypotheses, nothing about these cycles can be proved at the present time.

The hypothesis of Professor Franz Halberg, of the University of Minnesota, a man recognized as the world's leading authority on circadian cycles, is of considerable interest. Opening the skulls of rats, he removed as much of the brain as was compatible with the maintaining of life. As a result of these experiments, he learned that the twenty-four-hour activity changes in the body temperatures, basal metabolisms, functioning of the liver and kidneys, and secreting of hormones gradually failed to agree with each other.

The cerebral cortex of the brain or the pineal body senses the rotation of the earth and employs this environmental factor in controlling the functions of the various organs and vessels of the body. In Dr. Halberg's experiments, this part of the brains of the rats was removed. Consequently, when the controlling device was no longer present, each of the organs of the body began to operate according to its own individual rhythm. In biological-rhythms terminology, this is called free-running-system research.

During three billion years of evolution, the operations of the bodily organs have been regulated to conform roughly with the twenty-four-hour cycle. (Of course this differs somewhat with the individual animal; but, in man, the cycle is maintained with a variation of range of plus or minus two hours.) The system does not operate with clockwork accuracy. It has been experimentally proved, however, that the cerebral cortex and such glands as the pineal function to reduce time differentials in the operations of these rhythms. In other words, it is the cerebral cortex and its adjunct that function to make automatic corrections to match the actions of the organs to the circadian cycle. In terms of ordinary clocks, then, the cerebral cortex functions as pendulum and balance wheel.

The influences of the individual cycles of the bodily organs sometimes disrupt the general system of automatic regulation. When this happens, two systems interfere with each other. This produces a result that in terms of physics is comparable to the humming phenomenon that occurs when two sounds of different frequencies interfere with each other. For example, the overlapping of sounds of 230 and 240 hertz produces a ten-hertz hum; that is, a cycle twenty times greater in amplitude than the lower of the frequencies causing it. Of course, the phenomenon in living organisms is much more complicated than this.

The cyclic occurrence of a similar interference phenomenon in the metabolic system and the roughly one-month duration of the cycle is highly plausible and reasonable from the standpoint of biological rhythm.

The energy involved in the humming phenomenon is not great; consequently, the hum itself sometimes goes unperceived. Similarly, biorhythm conditions are not as clearly apparent as the twenty-four-hour circadian cycle. For this reason, they are often overlooked. In many instances, a person does not become aware of them unless he consults a calendar. Though strictly speaking different, undeniably the awareness of these cycles to an extent resembles autosuggestion.

The important thing is that the cycle I have been comparing to the hum caused by the interference of two different frequencies produces caution days in which the human individual is susceptible to illness, accident, and even death. The most reasonable way to strive for maximum human happiness is to accept the importance of this cycle and to take positive steps to avoid the dangers inherent in certain days. For this reason, I advocate the widest possible application of the system based on biorhythm.

In addition to the circadian cycle of the sun (or the rotation of the earth), the influence of the moon is thought to establish a roughly monthly cycle of physical and mental change. Dr. Curt Richter, of the Johns Hopkins University, in Baltimore, has partly proved the existence of a moon-related monthly cycle in both men and women. This cycle is totally unrelated to the menstrual cycle.

Dr. Richter insists that the existence of the lunar cycle in human beings, rats, monkeys, and other animals suggests that the cycle was established in the earliest stages of evolution. In the way that the light of the sun has created a twenty-four-hour cycle, so the light of the moon has created a monthly cycle. He adds that, during the process of evolution, the influence of the moon gradually weakened and the monthly biological cycle faded. Nonetheless, it has remained an important potential influential power in relation to human actions and bodily functions.

At the time of its birth, the moon, like the earth in the same age, was a flaming mass. But it died quickly without producing a biological system that reached the sophistication of the human animal. Dr. Richter says, however, that there may well have been a phase in biological evolution on earth in which the moon had as great —or greater—an influence on earthly animals as the sun. In terms of biological common sense, I agree with Dr. Richter.

Using rats, Dr. Richter has performed many experiments on social stresses and has written splendid papers that have won him worldwide fame. At an international symposium held in London in 1967, on the nature of hormones in connection with human activities, he reported on monthly cycles in many of the common diseases. His coverage included such things as schizophrenia, melancholia, epilepsy, hysteria, neurosis, hemophilia, eye trouble, and hundreds more.

The information made public at the fifth conference of the International Society for Biological Rhythms, held in Stockholm, in 1955, by Dr. Hilmar Heckert, of Berlin, was highly interesting because of the research he has done in the influence of the cycle of the moon on human life and death. He presented significant statistics showing that human births drop by about one-third in conjunction with the full and new moons, whereas human deaths increase by about 10 percent in connection with the new moon.

In attempting to ascertain the optimum approach to adopt toward a field of scientific study in which so many basics are unknown, I should like to mention a point of maximum importance made in a series of lectures on "Man Adapting" by the noted specialist Dr. René Dubos, of the Rockefeller Medical Institute. The gist of his message is contained in the following quotation: "Primitive man explains natural phenomena with magic; when we are confronted with the inexplicable we too often fall back on mysticism in somewhat more sophisticated language. . . . to which I can only answer that emphasizing the existence of unknowns or mysteries is not the same thing as believing in ghosts. To invoke ghosts constitutes a claim of explanation, whereas what I have tried to do is to call attention to phenomena that are certainly of importance to human welfare, yet are grossly neglected by medical science."

Even within the narrow field of biorhythm, there are mystical things that we do not understand. But this is no reason to invoke ghosts. Since it has been proved that it can be of service to human society, biorhythm deserves enthusiastic study and application.

The way biorhythm is applied varies with the country in question. The Germans and the Swiss, who are fond of philosophy and theory, are enthusiastic about it. The people of the Latin countries, who are more concerned with moods, and the practical and machine-oriented Americans pay less attention to it. I believe that the Japanese can make important contributions to the development and use of biorhythm and the behavioral science.

Human Birth

Rhythm for the human race is composed of the alternation of generations of reproductive and somatic cells. Biorhythm and the three PSI cycles begin at the instant of birth. It is important to acquire a certain amount of general information about the development of the embryo from the initial stages of pregnancy to the time of birth and about the drama of childbirth itself. Such knowledge is a basis for detailed understanding of biorhythm.

The flow of development that ends in the sophisticated organism called the human being begins with the sperm cell and the ovum. For animals of the complexity of man, virgin birth is an impossibility. On the other hand, reproduction does not invariably require sexual intercourse between male and female. Artificial insemination can be, and indeed is, used to produce pregnancy. There is even talk of the future use of artificial wombs for the development of human embryos. In other words, the era in which sexual intercourse can be the sole constituent of sexual education is passing.

Nonetheless, it is easy for insemination to occur during sexual intercourse between male and female. The sperm cell passes into the womb from the vagina, moves along a Fallopian tube, and there encounters an ovum descending along the tube. When this happens, the sperm cell enters the ovum; and insemination takes place.

The male testes constantly produce sperm cells. But the case is different with the ovaries, which produce ova only at about the middle part of the menstrual cycle at the stimulation of the luteinizing hormone secreted by the pituitary gland. Specialists call this process ovulation. The ovum passes downward along one of the Fallopian tubes. Generally pregnancy occurs when the ovum encounters sperm cells during this passage.

The fertilized ovum then passes into the womb, where it takes root on the womb wall. At first the connection between the two is very small, but it grows as the ovum absorbs nourishment from the female body. By about the third or fourth month of pregnancy, it has developed into a fully formed placenta. Until the placenta is formed, miscarriages can occur with relative ease. Furthermore, the embryo can be aborted in this early stage with less danger to the mother.

The placenta, which has a very special makeup, produces various hormones. In addition, it takes oxygen and nutrients from the mother's blood and passes them to the embryo and returns carbon dioxide and waste products from the circulation system of the embryo to the mother's bloodstream. The blood circulations of the mother and the embryo are not the same. Each organism has its own heart and its own circulation system; the two are connected by means of the special system of blood vessels in the chorion.

Cell division begins at insemination. In about one month, the ovum, which was originally about the size of a pinhead, has grown to about fingernail size. At this stage, the embryo resembles a seahorse.

By the third month of pregnancy the embryo has achieved something like human shape and has a total length of about two centimeters. With the completion of the placenta, the growth rate of the embryo accelerates. By the fourth month, the embryo is eleven centimeters long and much closer in appearance to a normal human being. It now moves with freedom in the amniotic fluids; the mother feels this as motion in her womb. The embryo continues to develop until, by the ninth month, it is approximately fifty centimeters long and weighs about three kilograms. The time of birth is approaching.

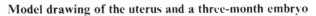

Model drawing of the uterus and a three-month embryo

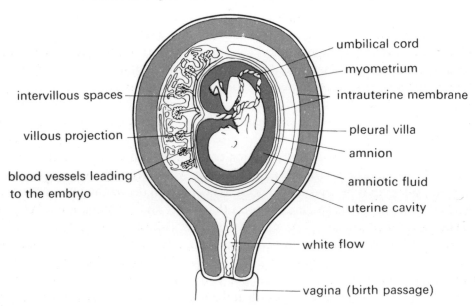

intervillous spaces

villous projection

blood vessels leading
to the embryo

umbilical cord

myometrium

intrauterine membrane

pleural villa

amnion

amniotic fluid

uterine cavity

white flow

vagina (birth passage)

Labor parturition, or the mechanical aspect of childbirth, begins with labor pains, the first stage of which is the rhythmical contraction of the muscles of the womb. The contractions continue until the uteral cervix is open and the head of the embryo has been forced out. In an initial childbirth, this process usually lasts from ten to sixteen hours. The second phase involves the passage of the child through the birth passage between the uteral cervix and the vagina and completely outside the body of the mother. This is usually accomplished in two hours after the opening of the birth passage. The third phase is the release of the placenta from the uteral wall and its passage along the birth canal and out of the mother's body. This usually takes from five to ten minutes.

After birth, the doctor or midwife at once cleans the infant's mouth and waits for it to make its first cry. Ordinarily this occurs immediately. If it does not, the doctor holds the infant upside down and lightly taps it twice or three times on the back. If this treatment fails, an oxygen mask must be used to initiate artificial respiration.

The initial cry, the infant's first contact with the outside world, is of the greatest importance because, until it is made, the baby is still relying on placental circulation; that is, it cannot supply oxygen from the air to its lungs. In other words, it is unable to support life in the outside world. If no throbbing motion is observed in the umbilical cord the midwife ties and cuts it, leaving about seven or eight centimeters beyond the navel.

Physiologically, the first cry of the baby is stimulated by the cessation of the oxygen supply that, till this time, has been supported by placental circulation of blood. The stimulation of a joint shortage of oxygen and an accumulation of carbon dioxide alters respiration and blood circulation. Before this time, blood has been flowing directly from the right auricle of the heart, through the oval foramen in the septum between the auricles, into the left auricle. With the natural closing of the oval foramen in the septum, blood flows from the right auricle to the right chamber and from there to the pulmonary trunk and to the capillaries in the lungs. There it comes into contact with the air from outside, takes in oxygen, and travels through the pulmonary vein to the left auricle of the heart. In other words, this is the first step in normal, healthy pulmonary circulation. It is believed that the stimulus accompanying this respiration is a causatory factor in the accelerated development of nerves that takes place for about two months following birth.

The first cry, the change from placental to pulmonary circulation, is the most dramatic moment in the history of individual human life. Neither the advent of puberty nor natural death can compare with it. Though it is dramatic in itself, natural death is not as sudden and abrupt an event because the various parts of the body die one by one after the heart or the brain has ceased to function.

Naegle's law for the prediction of the day of birth is most reliable. It calls for adding seven days to the last menstruation and then subtracting three months from that. Although only 10 percent of infants are born on exactly the day predicted by this method, 75 percent are born within two weeks on either side of that date.

In his book *Biologische Fragmente zu einer Lehre vom Menschen*, the Swiss professor at Basel University Adolf Portmann has said that human beings are born very soon from the physiological standpoint. By this he means that, in comparison with the offspring of other mammals, the human infant is immature at birth. If the human infant waited to reach a stage of maturity comparable to those of other mammals at birth, it would remain in the womb for twenty-one months. Consequently, the impact of birth on the human infant must be much greater than that on infants of other mammals.

The Role of Hormones

From the standpoint of medical balance, the autonomic nervous system and the endocrine system, which is constantly controlled by it, are of the greatest importance. Classical medicine referred to the relation between the two as homeostasis, but more recently the word *homeokinesis* has come into popular use. The pituitary gland is a center of dynamic equilibrium. Unless it functions properly, menstrual irregularities occur. It is especially interesting from the biorhythm standpoint that Dr. Curt Richter has reported the effectiveness of the thyroid hormones in the treatment of cyclic diseases.

The autonomic nervous system and the endocrine system work together to prevent irregularities in body cells, tissues, vessels, and other systems, and to enable the body to deal with stimuli and stresses from the outside environment. The balance maintained between the systems is a dynamic one of constant living flow. It extends from the level of the microscopic to the level of macroscopic observations. The condition of active balance between them suggests the Yin and Yang philosophy of Chinese medicine and the true and false symptoms of illness in Western medicine. It can be interpreted as feedback from the increasing and decreasing amounts of hormones secreted. This phenomenon is called homeokinesis, or simply dynamic equilibrium.

The study of the relation between the nervous and endocrine systems is correlative physiology. Progress in this study has influenced research in biorhythm. Though it remains only hypothetical, the cyclic action of biorhythm is thought to be activated by hormones. The menstrual cycle seems to be one factor substantiating this hypothesis. Unfortunately, even the most sophisticated modern scientific knowledge is not able to define why the menstrual cycle should be twenty-nine days long on the average. All that can be said is that experience teaches us it is that long. And, as I have said earlier, we cannot say why the biorhythm cycles are twenty-three, twenty-eight, and thirty-three days long.

We can say that the menstrual cycle results from the dynamic balance of the operations of more than five hormones: three produced by the anterior lobe of the pituitary gland—the gonadotropic, or the follicle-stimulating; the luteinizing and the luteotrophic hormones—plus estrogens and progesterone produced by the ovaries. Furthermore, the balanced operation of these hormones affects the nervous condition and countless other factors. For instance, it is not unusual for women to miss a menstrual period because of moving to a new house or beginning a new job. Sometimes such dramatic things as spurious pregnancy occur.

Dr. Richter performed experiments in which he removed the ovaries of female monkeys and the testes of male monkeys and learned that such operations had no effect on biorhythm cycles. This proved that the hormones secreted by the gonads are unrelated to biorhythm and that the menstrual cycle is independent of them.

The adrenocorticotrophic hormone, produced by the anterior lobe of the pituitary gland, stimulates the adrenal cortex to secrete the cortisone group of hormones, famous because of the stress theory of Dr. Hans Selye. These and the catecholamine group (adrenalin and noradrenalin), which is closely related to the autonomic nervous system, provide important sources of energy for the circadian cycles. From the standpoint of the work of Dr. Halberg, the participation of the adrenal gland, which is governed by the pituitary gland, and of the autonomic nervous system is of major importance.

Dr. Richter, on the other hand, claims that, not only in the cases of human beings, but in those of other animals as well, there is abundant data to suggest important participation on the part of the hormones produced by the thyroid gland: thyroxine and triiodothyronine. But there is a dynamic equilibrium in the amounts of these hormones produced because of stimulation of the thyroid gland by the thyrostimulating hormone, which is secreted by the pituitary gland. Reduction of the functioning of the thyroid gland aggravates those diseases described by Dr. Richter as cyclic. Conversely, stimulation of the thyroid gland can cause improvements in these sicknesses in both human beings and other animals.

I am especially interested in this because the level of functioning of the thyroid glands of the Japanese is on an average lower than the level in Western peoples. It seems unlikely at the present that this is a hereditary matter. The low level of thyroid functioning among the Japanese is probably related to diet. Iodine, natrium, and potassium are required to stimulate the secretion of the thyroid hormones. Analyses of the Japanese diet show that ample amounts of these substances are eaten. The problem lies in the excessively salty foods the Japanese eat with their staple, rice. These salts tend to cause the valuable minerals needed for thyroid-hormone production to be passed out through the kidneys. For this reason, adjustments must be made in the amounts of salts taken by people who are easily influenced by biorhythm.

The relation between the nervous system and the endocrine system is like that between the tortoise and the hare in the famous fable. The nervous system acts quickly but tends to be lazy. The hormones act slowly but steadily. It is physiological common sense, then, to assume that the hormones form the basis of the monthly biorhythmic cycles.

From the preceding discussion, it is possible to deduce the following: the pituitary gland and the adrenal hormone system or the pituitary gland and the thyroid hormone system—acting either together or separately—establish biorhythm. The amplitude of change in the rhythm is at most about half that of the changes in the yearly seasonal rhythms, or no more than 5 percent. This falls within the permissible margin of error in modern techniques for measuring hormones. Some of the devices marketed today for biorhythm estimations mislead by claiming greater hormone variation than this and cause persons relying on them to indulge in unscientific autosuggestion. Much of the anxiety experienced on caution days is nervous and not directly hormone-controlled at all. Dramatic illnesses, deaths, accidents, and suicides may have been caused by nervous reactions to such mistaken approaches to biorhythm.

Combination with Autogenic Training

The biorhythm that I have developed in Japan is not fatalistic. It is based on the idea of autogenic training, which must now be explained. In the following section, I make special use of data connected with the medical research of Dr. Wolfgang Luthe. My version of biorhythm incorporates elements of ancient oriental systems like Yoga and Zen.

Although autogenic training, developed in the 1920's by Dr. Johannes Heinrich Schultz, has a history nearly as long as that of biorhythm, it is said to have been introduced into Japan no earlier than 1952. After the formation of the Society for Psychosomatic Medicine, in 1960, by Dr. Torijiro Ikemi, of Kyushu University, interest in this kind of academic training spread rapidly in Japan. The speed of its growth in popularity may be accounted for by the points it has in common with Yoga and Zen. Indeed, Dr. Schultz said that these oriental training systems provided hints for the evolution of autogenic training.

I realized this relation because of my studies in stress theories and long advocated the possibility of combining biorhythm and autogenic training. But I was unable to put this idea into practice and thus produce actual results until I began work on accident reduction in commercial organizations.

In 1963, Dr. Kraus Thomas, one of Dr. Schultz's leading disciples and the director of the Suicide Prevention Center in Berlin, came to Japan on his way to the United States and gave a number of lectures on autogenic training and suicide prevention. As both a medical doctor and a theologian, Dr. Thomas spoke in a highly convincing way that made a great impression on all of us. Because there are many written commentaries on the work of Dr. Schultz and Dr. Ikemi, there is no need to go further into the subject in detail here.

In general, autogenic training is divisible into short- and long-term programs. In the short program, the person conducts five-minute sessions twice daily—morning and evening. In these sessions, he gives himself suggestions related to the various parts of the body. For instance, he thinks as follows: my right arm is heavy; my left arm is warm; I am breathing comfortably, and my heart is beating calmly; my stomach is warm; and so on. He concludes the session by suggesting to himself that his forehead is cool. From two to four months of such sessions constitute short-term training. The long-term course consists of the same kind of training extended over a period ranging from six months to three years. Tests made on brain waves to examine the effectiveness of the training reveal various levels of difference. In 1960 and 1961, the Japanese Ministry of Education provided grants for study of the physiological effects of seated Zen meditation on brain waves, energy metabolism, respiration, pulse, and galvanic skin response. These studies showed that seated Zen meditation and long-term autogenic training have approximately the same effects.

Section of the brain on a line perpendicular to the forehead

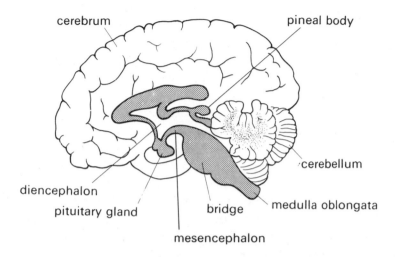

cerebrum

pineal body

cerebellum

diencephalon

pituitary gland

bridge

medulla oblongata

mesencephalon

The Canadian Dr. Wolfgang Luthe has proved that, from the standpoint of alterations in brain waves, the effect of autogenic training is different from that of the intermediate stage of sleep. Autogenic training greatly limits the activities of the reticular formation and the cortex. At the same time, it lowers the centrifugal activities of the thalamus and the cortex. In addition, it immediately causes functional variations in such of the nervous structures related to the reticular formation as the hyperthalamus, cerebellum, brain stems, and other nervous nuclei. Briefly put, the result of these influences is to stabilize the activity of body and mind.

In this respect, autogenic training produces a state resembling half-sleep; but people who have trained for a long time are able to extend this state into everyday life.

In terms of physiological changes, training lowers rectal temperatures, reduces skin temperatures and circulation, normalizes peristaltic action, lowers body temperature, normalizes electrocardiograph reactions, reduces the cholesterol level in the blood serum, and lowers respiration rates. Further, it is reported to have an effect on the endocrine system, which affects and balances physical and mental functioning.

In his investigations of autogenic training effects on two people, the Norwegian specialist Dr. R. Alnaes discovered that trainees with more than six months of experience maintain a lowered level of the adrenocortical hormone. This effect persisted wite the result that stress was lowered in the trainees.

Using protein-bound iodine as an indicator, Dr. Luthe conducted checks on the amounts of the adrenocortical hormone in patients. Dr. P. Polzien, of Würzburg University, conducted experiments on the basal metabolic rates of patients with hyperthyroidism (Graves's disease). In both cases, reductions were experienced by people who practiced autogenic training. Dr. Polzien discovered that patients who continued training were cured of the hyperthyroidal condition in from six months to a year. After eight years had passed, not a single patient had suffered a recurrence of hyperthyroidism.

The stress theory of Dr. Hans Selye is important; but it belongs to methods advocating low-tone control. Nonetheless, I must say here that his system seems to me to have much in common with Zen practices.

Dr. Ikemi has some interesting observations to make about the methods of world-famous psychological therapist Dr. Ainslie Meares, of Australia, in his preface to the Japanese edition of Meares's book *Relief Without Drugs*. Dr. Ikemi says that Dr. Meares's repetition of words like *natural* to patients whom he has succeeded in putting in a relaxed state is a way of halting the flood of thoughts that have been filling the patient's mind and of making him feel one with nature. In this way, he helps the patient attune his mental wave lengths to the rules of nature and discover that the youthful power for self-normalization and self-regulation exists within him.

Although I have concentrated on Dr. Schultz's autogenic training, there are other systems that can be called autogenic in a wider sense. For instance, Dr. Schultz says that he used as reference both Zen Buddhism and Yoga, which might be described as ancient oriental systems of autogenic training.

A word of practical advice is needed for those who suspect that a goal is necessary for training of this kind. A goal is necessary. By all means set one. If you are ill, practice autogenic training until you are cured. If you are a student studying for examinations, use autogenic training to help you. But, when you have achieved the original goal, immediately set another. Do not undertake autogenic training merely because it is the fashion. Have motivation. As I shall discuss later, motivation is of the utmost value. Having it helps prevent falling into the misunderstanding that biorhythm is fatalistic. It is because the combination of autogenic training, bio-rhythm, and motivation steers clear of fatalism that my system remains in close contact with ordinary daily living. This in turn is the reason why the system has made progress in Japan.

Motivation and Morale

The system that has been worked out in Japan is to combine a biorhythm calendar with autogenic training and to make sure that the person undergoing training has motivation. In this section I explain motivation from the standpoint of behavioral science and in relation to morale.

The system that I have developed into a behavioral science is not merely a copy of something imported from the West. In Western countries, biorhythm is largely passively interpreted as a fatalistic kind of fortune telling. I have basically revised the system by combining the study of biorhythm with autogenic training and have insisted on the provision of motivation. In this way, the system has become positive and goal-oriented.

My first hint for the modification of the system was the need for an improved biorhythm calendar (see p. 57). I placed emphasis on the caution days of the three PSI cycles and arranged the material so that it would be immediately understandable in its entirety. I made a large column for memoranda in the form of a schedule. Combining the daily PSI conditions with a diary in this way, instead of carrying them separately, meant that it would be possible to persevere in autogenic training automatically and effectively. This was the initial step in the development of a biorhythm science of behavior.

In my thirty and more years of study on problems of stress and fatigue, I have learned that, in discussing such subjects, it is always necessary to take morale into account. Without consideration of morale, all talk of antifatigue measures is pie in the sky, utterly unrelated to actuality. Without the morale element, biorhythm in Japan would not have developed into a behavioral science. For this reason, I include morale as one of the biorhythm basics.

I have been using the words *behavioral science* without explanation, even though some of my readers may not know their exact meaning. Pinning the meaning down is difficult. Even in the United States, where the expression originated, it is used in two senses: psychological and managerial. Nonetheless, behavioral science is important enough to be taught in public-health courses. For instance, Harvard University, one of my alma maters, has started a department and course in the subject.

Since I am a doctor, naturally I base my thought primarily on physiology and psychology. In addition, however, I have taught human ecology to health-center doctors for twenty-five years and have been the Japanese representative to the International Association for Suicide Prevention for the past twenty years. On the basis of my varied experience, I have evolved an interpretation of human behavior that is represented in the chart above. Human behavior may be approached from three angles: the sociocultural, the physiological-biochemical, and the psychological-autonomic. Any of these approaches can constitute a science of behavior.

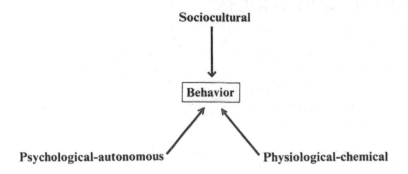

The value of biorhythm to behavioral science may be stated as follows: it is an individual technique for the unconscious establishment of a constructive morale as motivation by means of the introduction of conscious behavior into the realm of subconscious behavior by virtue of cyclic segmentation.

Motivation is of surprisingly great importance to human endurance and achievement. In a book I wrote on antifatigue measures in the information society, I related experiments conducted by a doctor at Harvard University on the effect of motivation on the ability to hang suspended. Hypnosis on a person who could normally hang from an iron bar for only fifty seconds enabled him to hang in the same fashion for seventy seconds. The promise of a reward of fifty dollars for a better record stimulated the same person to hang from the bar for two minutes.

To give another illustration, I might mention Bob who lives in the Boston suburbs. Ordinarily, he is allegedly able to run only twenty meters to catch the train. To catch the next-to-last train home at night, however, he is able to run forty, and to catch the last train, seventy meters. A strong motivating factor accounts for his vastly improved performance late at night. If he misses the last train, he must pay thirty dollars in taxi fare or stay in town only to face his wife's demand for a convincing explanation on the following day.

Whether we are aware of it or not, motivation is a powerful constructive morale element in our daily lives. This is why I insist on combining motivation with biorhythm and autogenic training.

For the sake of continued improvement of the behavioral science I have evolved around these elements, I myself have a very strong motivation. I have a deep desire to demonstrate my respect for life by striving to reduce its loss in traffic accidents through the application of this system. My motivation enables me to turn a deaf ear to critics who claim that the Japanese use of biorhythm to this end is no more than autosuggestion.

How to Relax

In busy, modern society, it is recognized that relaxing is a key to improved efficiency in work. In the case of biorhythm, too, the ability to relax greatly improves the overall effect of training.

One of the first experts to come to mind in connection with relaxation is Dr. Edmund Jacobson, of the Chicago Institute of Clinical Physiology. Dr. Jacobson studied under the world famous Dr. Walter B. Cannon, of Harvard. Dr. Cannon, whose achievements have won him immense general recognition, is especially noted for his work on pain, hunger, fear, and rage in cats. These words were used in his time to express the concept that today we lump together under the single word *stress*. One of Dr. Cannon's classic experiments was to put a cat in a cage and to allow dogs to walk freely around the imprisoned animal. Under such conditions, the cat's suprarenal gland secreted large amounts of adrenalin and noradrenalin to cause such physiological reactions as dilation of the pupils, frothing at the mouth, and erection of the fur. These emergency reactions announce to the body a state of extreme danger in which life may be at stake.

My honored teacher Dr. Hans Selye performed similar experiments on rats. He did not limit himself to psychological elements, but discovered that stress caused by heat, cold, and chemical poison also causes massive secretions of suprarenal cortex hormones. He called this the alarm reaction. Though it is less profound than emergency reactions, if prolonged, it can produce such diseases of adaptation as high blood pressure, stomach ulcers, and heart troubles.

Dr. Bibb Latané performed interesting experiments in connection with adrenalin. He created stress situations in rats by means of electric shocks and then taught the animals how to escape from the shock. He administered injections of adrenalin in three strengths to rats kept under these conditions and examined the effects of the shots on the rats' abilities to escape. He learned that adrenalin improves this ability and that smaller injections produce somewhat better effects than large ones. This suggests the condition athletes sometimes experience before an important match, when excitement builds up to so great a point that they are prevented from doing as well as usual.

The medulla of the suprarenal gland contains ten milligrams of adrenalin; a sudden injection of two milligrams is sufficient to induce death by shock. It is easy to see that disturbances in the regulation of this hormone on days that are critical in terms of biorhythm could have the gravest effects.

Psychologically induced stress causes hormone reactions that last much longer than might be expected, as was demonstrated by Dr. John W. Mason, of the American Army Hospital. Dr. Mason created avoidance-conditioned stress in monkeys and examined the durations of effects on hormones. He found that secretion of adrenalin was restored to normal in two days. Secretions of noradrenalin, the suprarenal cortex hormones, and the thyroid hormones, on the other hand, increased in volume after the first day and did not return to normal until a week had passed. In connection with this, the following advice from Dr. Selye ought to be born in mind always:

"It is not easy to tune down when you have reached your stress-quota. Many more people are the helpless slaves of their own stressful activities than of alcohol. Besides, simple rest is no cure-all. Activity and rest must be judiciously balanced, and every person has his own characteristic requirements for rest and activity. To lie motionless in bed all day is no relaxation for an active man.

"All work and no play is certainly harmful for anyone at any age; but then, what is work and what is play? Fishing is relaxing play for the business executive, but it is hard work for the professional fisherman. The former can go fishing to relax, but the latter will have to do something else, or simply take a rest, in order to relax."

As our way of living becomes increasingly active, the ability to relax becomes increasingly important. The combination of biorhythm and autogenic training can help. To illustrate my point, I shall return to the work of Dr. Jacobson and relate an episode about a tennis player that he includes in his book *Introduction to Relaxation.*

The player had his first consultation on this matter in 1936 and became convinced that learning how to relax would improve his efficiency. He had become aware of tension during tennis matches brought on by excessive awareness of the spectators. He received instructions on how to relax and practiced what he was taught daily. He found that his tennis skills improved to the point where his coach noticed greater relaxation in his swing and rhythm. In 1940, this man did exceptionally well in tennis. Many years after going to work for a shipbuilding firm, he continued to practice relaxation training; and, at the age of forty-nine, in 1950, he had the blood-pressure count of a man of twenty.

For tense people, relaxation by means of repeated autogenic training is most important, especially on caution days. The following mini-Zen session helps achieve the desired result.

1. After loosening the clothes—especially belts, corsets, neckties, and other binding articles—sit straight in a chair and lightly close your eyes. Easy chairs and reclining chairs will not do, because the back must be held straight and the chin must be pulled in. The knees must be at right angles, and the soles of the feet must be flat on the floor.

2. Raise your arms straight over your head. Knit the fingers of both hands together. Tensing the fingers, swing both arms to the rear. Repeat slowly three times.

36

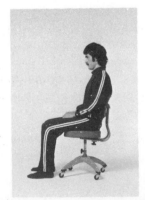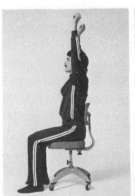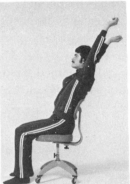

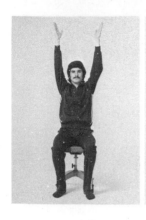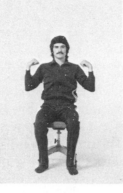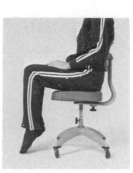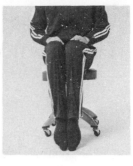

3. Spreading the fingers of both hands, lower and raise your arms at right angles to the side. Repeat slowly three times.

4. Point your toes and raise your heels well from the floor. Repeat slowly three times.

5. Begin breathing so that you employ the muscles of your abdomen. Inhale for three seconds and exhale for seven. Leave a comfortable interval between inhalation and the initiation of exhalation. Ordinarily, it is possible to establish this rhythm after four or five breaths. Concentrate on the breathing rhythm.

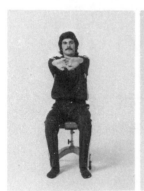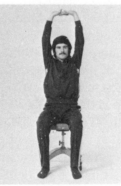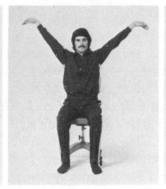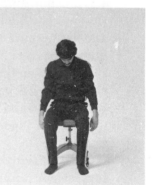

Interlock the fingers of both hands and stretch your arms out in front of you. Keeping your elbows straight, raise your arms above your head.

Open your hands and swing your arms in circles to the side. Relax your entire body.

6. There is no need to be absolutely accurate in counting; but, after about ten breaths, roughly three minutes should have elapsed.

7. Say to yourself, "I'm very comfortable now."

This concludes the mini-Zen session. You do not need to say the sentence aloud at first. But, if you repeat this mini-Zen session daily for a number of days, you will come to want to say it aloud. On biorhythm caution days, repeat this mini-Zen session four or five times throughout the morning, afternoon, and evening. Each session lasts only three minutes.

I should like to say a word about the importance of loosening the clothing, especially the necktie, which is in itself a symbol of tension. I have shirts made in a fashion that permits easy relaxation. Since not everyone has such shirts, remember that leaving the necktie tied tight greatly reduces the effectiveness of the mini-Zen session.

The Science of Timing

Timing is of the essence, as obstetricians and other people who work constantly with the great drama of birth know well. In this section, I begin with a quotation from the enlightening writings of the Canadian doctor Marion Hilliard. Then I discuss the concept of *Biotakt*, a main element in the thought of the philosopher Dr. Ludwig Klages. Finally, I discuss catecholeamine hormones and their relation to the control of animal behavior.

In connection with the wider meaning of biorhythm and with the narrower meaning of the PSI theory, I often talk in terms of the science of timing because, objectively analyzed, biorhythm is a matter of the skillful or inept application of timing. The book *A Woman Doctor Looks at Love and Life* by Dr. Marion Hilliard, professor and head of the Obstetrics Department of the Toronto Woman's Medical University, was a major stimulus in my decision to combine the science of timing with biorhythm. The book became a best seller immediately after initial publication in 1957 and has been translated into six languages, including Japanese. Here I should like to quote a passage from the chapter entitled "Timing and Rhythm":

"I believe in timing. It is crystallized for me in the moment of greatness that an athlete like Mickey Mantle knows for that fraction of time when his bat meets the ball squarely and sends it out of the park. This is true timing—the health and animal instinct of a superb athlete performing perfectly at the time and place best suited to him.

"All individuals must find this kind of timing. In that lovely movie *Lili*, the girl says, 'There is a time for growing up, there is a time for going to school, there is a time for falling in love.' This timing process can't be rushed or the whole pattern of life is jostled. It must be taken with fluid grace, one step at a time. This is the beginning of wisdom.

"Timing has its own rhythm. In each life there is a time, clearly defined by nature in the extra vigor of the young, for striving and ambition; there is an ebb time for tranquility. There is a time for passion and a time for contentment. The reckless ones who try to jar the rhythm and look for peace when it is too soon or accomplishment when it is too late can only be shattered."

Perhaps it is her experience in dealing with the drama of birth that has enabled Dr. Hilliard to write in a lyrical way that reminds me of the music of Frederic Chopin. She is certainly of one mind with me about timing. As I said at the opening of this book, the source of all life for the three and one-half billion people on earth is the correct timing of the encounter between the ovum and the sperm cell.

For a more learned and objective interpretation of the relation between biorhythm and timing, I shall turn to the work of Dr. Ludwig Klages and his book *Vom Wesen des Rhythmus* (The Essence of Rhythm). After taking his degree from the University of Munich, Dr. Klages decided not to enter the teaching profession and to devote himself entirely to philosophical writing in the field of phenomenology. In *Vom Wesen des Rhythmus*, which was first published in 1923, Dr. Klages says that rhythm is the orderly repetition of temporal phenomenological elements and always belongs to the world of phenomena. He cites the remark by the Greek philosopher Heraclitus to the effect that it is impossible to enter the same river twice. Not only will the water in the river have flowed by, but also the individual human being will have aged to an extent and will no longer be the same. To understand this clearly it is only necessary to compare the ways of looking at the world of a five-year-old child and a seventy-year-old man.

Dr. Klages adds that, in connection with the phenomenon of rhythm, we human beings attempt to make psychological segmentations from which time measures (*Takt* in German) come into being. It is precisely because our minds are motivated to establish divisions and regularity that we are aware of rhythm as measures of time. Rhythm is a constantly renewing, general-life phenomenon, whereas *Takt* is a repetitive psychological activity on the part of the individual human being attempting to conform to rhythm. Consequently, in introducing into behavioral science the PSI theory accompanied by motivation, I have moved from the world of pure biorhythm into the world of *Biotakt*.

Dr. Klages gives a strikingly pertinent illustration when he speaks of two excellent dancers, one of whom was continually irritated and the other of whom was always cheerful. When the two danced together, the cheerful one always seemed more skillful. The irritated one, by attempting to suppress the rhythm within natural life phenomena, appeared less skillful but, as might be expected, relaxed and danced better after having a small amount of alcohol. What Dr. Klages has to say proves the validity of combining behavioral science with something like Dr. Schultz's autogenic training by means of biorhythm (more accurately *Biotakt*) as an intermediary.

Before concluding this chapter, I have a few more remarks to make on the interesting relations between hormones and human behavior that were proved as the result of the research of Dr. Ulf von Euler, of the University Institute of Karolinska, in Sweden. For his work in this field, Dr. Euler was awarded the Nobel Prize for physiology in 1970. The relation between hormones and behavior was discovered as a result of investigations of the differences between carnivorous and herbivorous animals.

In addition to the suprarenal cortex hormones, researched by Dr. Selye, the suprarenal body produces hormones originating from its medulla: adrenalin and noradrenalin, which in terms of embryology arise from the same sources as the nerves. There is no difference between the two in terms of the presence or absence of the methyl group. Their functions, however, do differ. Adrenalin, sometimes referred to as the surprise hormone, accelerates the pulse and causes palpitations. Noradrenalin, on the other hand, reduces the pulse rate and has a completely relaxing effect. These two hormones have contrary effects on human behavior, as has been clearly shown by the work of Dr. Fred Elmadjian, of the Worcester Foundation for Experimental Biology, in the United States, and by Dr. Daniel H. Funkenstein, of

Harvard. The extrovert, who is quick to display anger, is dominated by noradrenalin; and the introvert, who shows surprise in a negative way, is adrenalin dominated. Hopefully, biorhythm study, employing autogenic training, will be able to develop a way to control and balance the secretion of these two hormones.

Part 2 | Technical Development

Determining Caution Days

Dr. Fliess spoke of days on which episodes are likely to occur. Because of my emphasis on morale and a positive approach to behavioral science, I prefer terms like *days demanding caution* or *caution days* since they suggest that, with caution, the threatened episode can be averted. The biorhythm system used in Japan places great importance on caution days, their accurate calculation, and the way they are represented in charts and personal records.

Dr. Fliess learned that the timing of the individual's biorhythm is determined at the instant of birth. Later a number of engineers, attempted to verify the physical cycle of 23 days and the sensitivity cycle of 28 days on the basis of the 23 chromosomes of the human being and the average human gestation period of 280 days. But, since this is biologically only a coincidence, they failed to provide a theoretical basis for biorhythm with this approach.

Reasons for this failure were presented by the pediatrician Dr. Theodor Hellbruegge, of Munich University, at a conference of the International Association for Biological Rhythms held in 1960, at Cold Spring Harbor, New York. He showed that there is a definitive difference between the circadian variations occurring in the pulse rates of the embryo and the mother. Whereas the mother demonstrates clear adult circadian changes, the embryo maintains a constant pulse rate of 100 per minute for all 24 hours of the day (see graph below). Circadian changes in the

Changes in the pulse rates of the mother and the embryo

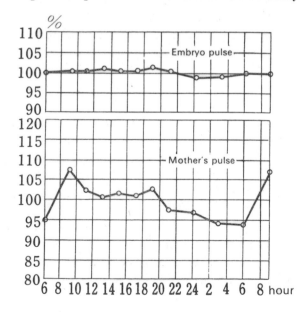

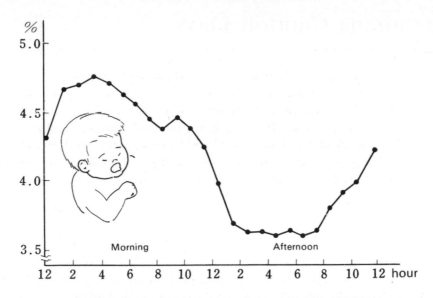

Distribution of the times of the day at which children
are born (601, 222 births between 1848 and 1960)

newborn infant's pulse develop very gradually. At one month after birth, they have
barely appeared; but, at the third month, an up-and-down variation range about
one-third as great as that of an adult has developed. The same phenomenon occurs
in relation to circadian changes in body temperature. This seems to be an expression
of the biological rule that the embryo develops independent of the time factor that is
a causative element in the establishment of rhythm. Furthermore, almost no infants
are born on the two-hundred-and-eightieth day. This figure for human gestation is
only an average. Experience shows, however, that days of birth are likely to occur
on the mothers' caution days. It would seem likely that engineers who maintained
the theory stated earlier were incorrectly linking the tendency for infants to be born
on their mothers' caution days with a supposed proof of embryonic rhythm.

Indeed, it is probable that the conditions of the mother, not those of the embryo,
determine the date of birth. A biological rule can be deduced from this; from the
tendency of mothers to deliver early in first childbirths; and from the frequency with
which nutrition, working conditions, and emotional stress cause premature births.

Furthermore, there are clear circadian variations in the times of childbirth. At the
1961 meeting of the International Conference for Biological Rhythms, Dr. I. H.
Kaiser, of the Obstetrics Department of Utah University, presented a report on times
of births of 600,000 infants born from 1848 to 1960. Results of his statistical studies
are shown in the graph above. They seem to endorse an old tradition to the effect
that babies are usually born at night. He showed that numbers of births begin to
increase after midnight, reach a peak at three in the morning, decline thereafter, reach
a low from noon until seven in the evening, and begin to pick up again after eight.

On the average, births tend to take place after midnight and in the early morning.
To be accurate, the twelve hours before birth and the twelve hours after birth con-

The three biorhythm conditions

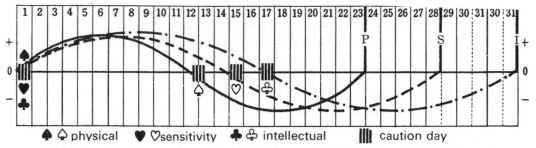

♠ ♤ physical   ♥ ♡ sensitivity   ♣ ♧ intellectual   ▓ caution day

Both this indication figure and Biocycle Mini are independently patented and copyrighted in 1974. If colored, P is blue, S is red, and I is green by the standard of Japan Biorhythm Laboratory.

stitute the first caution day. In other words, the first caution day of the individual human can often fall on two calendar days. But, since this makes calculations difficult, the calendar day of birth is usually taken as the basis for further figuring. For example, for a person born on October 1, the twenty-four hours of October 1 are considered the first caution day. In other words, the calculation is based on the premise that the child was born at noon, in which case his first caution day would in fact consist of the twelve hours from midnight to noon and the twelve hours from noon to midnight.

Recently, people in the field of biorhythm have adopted the policy of referring to what Dr. Fliess called episode days as caution days. In Germany and Switzerland, the terms *cycle day* (*Periodische Tage*) and *half-cycle day* (*Halbperiodische Tage*) persist. They have their value. If the caution days are represented in the form of a graph (p. 45), it will be seen that there is one at the first day of the cycle and one in the middle of the cycle; that is, two caution days in each cycle. In terms of the biological law pertaining to energy, these two caution days are the reverse of each other: the first is a day of instability and need for caution because of a transition from negative to positive energy; and the second is unstable because of a switch from positive to negative energy. In German and Swiss terminology, the first is the cycle day and the second the half-cycle day. As will be seen later, when I discuss the death dates of famous people, physical episodes tend to occur with greater frequency on half-cycle days.

But, unless purely mathematical calculations and biological considerations are kept completely separate in dealing with biorhythm, serious mistakes can arise. Using the assumption that the person who was born at noon, the German method considers this day the first caution day for all three cycles: physical, sensitivity, and intellectual. Since the physical cycle is twenty-three days long, the next caution day will fall during the twenty-four hours between the afternoon of the twelfth and the morning of the thirteenth. This day will be what the Germans and the Swiss call the half-cycle day. Since the sensitivity cycle is twenty-eight days, the half-cycle day will occur conveniently on the fifteenth. The intellectual cycle, like the physical one, will not divide in half as conveniently; consequently, the intellectual caution day (half-cycle) will fall from the afternoon of the seventeenth to the morning of the eighteenth.

This is the mathematical way of making determinations, but in biological terms, episodes merely tend to concentrate on caution days. Ultimately they must be represented by a bell curve of the kind devised by the statistician Adolphe Quételet. The one below shows on-the-job accidents that occurred on the Japan National Railways in 1968. The peak is seen at the caution day, and accidents sharply decrease on the right and left of it. The solid line shows serious accidents or deaths. The broken line represents minor accidents. The grave accidents show a much greater concentration on the caution day. As I shall explain in further detail later, serious occurrences are more remarkable in terms of biorhythm. This is important in accident prevention.

As should be clear, the exact time of birth is vital to the calculation of caution days. If you notice that your caution days as worked out mathematically do not coincide with the days on which you experience actual episodes, you may not have had accurate information about the time of your birth. Keep careful memoranda of things that happen to you, plot them, and make adjustments in your mathematically calculated caution days as is needed. It is important that each individual keep careful personal memoranda and not rely entirely on simple positive-negative curve graphs or on computers sold for biorhythm calculations.

Biorhythm distribution of on-the-job accidents

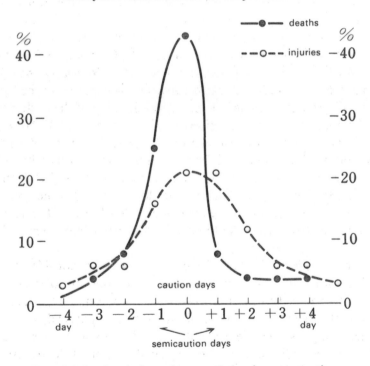

This distribution is based on statistics for twenty-three accidental deaths on the Japan National Railways in the first six months of 1968 and thirty-three injuries in the Tokyo Track Maintenance Department between 1966 and 1968. (From a biorhythm report on the Tokyo Track Maintenance Department by Haruo Miyake.)

Basic Biorhythm Calculations

The analysis of Dr. Fliess on episodes of illness showed that biorhythm begins at the moment of birth and continues in three cycles—twenty-three-day physical cycle, twenty-eight-day sensitivity cycle, and thirty-three-day intellectual cycle. As biological rule, they automatically adjust themselves in the long ran and make scrupulous calculations about them possible. Their basic calculations are explained here.

The charts used for calculating biorhythm of the wanted day are various, and many of them have been used to meet different purposes. At the initial phases of Dr. Fliess's research, a basic method of calculation was employed; it was primitive but is still useful in determining whether or not the days on which episodes occur are actually pertinent to the physical, sensitivity, and intellectual caution days. Of course, it requires more time than the easy calculation methods and involves a greater risk of error. But for the sake of deepening the reader's understanding of biorhythm, I shall offer a simple example of its application.

Person A was born on May 1, 1967. I shall use the primitive method to calculate his biorhythm condition on May 2, 1977, when he had just turned ten years of age. His tenth year ended on April 30, and he began a new year of his life on May 1. On May 2, he had been alive 3,655 days: $365 \times 10 + 3$ (for leap years) $+2$ (two days in May of the eleventh year)$=3,655$. These 3,655 days are his total days of life on May 2, 1977. The next step is to divide this figure by the numbers of days in the three cycles and to calculate the fractions.

$3,655 \div 23 = 158$ and a fraction (physical cycle 21)
$3,655 \div 28 = 130$ and a fraction (sensitivity cycle 15)
$3,655 \div 33 = 110$ and a fraction (intellectual cycle 25)

In other words, he is in the twenty-first day of his physical cycle, the fifteenth day of his sensitivity cycle, and the twenty-fifth day of his intellectual cycle. The sensitivity cycle is at a caution day (*Halbperiodische Tage* or half-period day), and the physical and intellectual cycles are in negative phases.

Once this basic method of calculation is understood, it is easier to design a simpler one. The date of birth consists of a year and a day of the month. My Tatai Tables A and B (see pp. 139–143) give the characteristic values for these. From the time of birth, each day has a physical cycle number from one to twenty-three, a sensitivity cycle number from one to twenty-eight, and an intellectual cycle number from one to thirty-three.

In this way, an A and a B chart can be determined, and then a C chart—for the given year and month—is established by a special calculation. It become possible to work out calculations on the basis of two-digit figures to simplify finding PSI conditions for any day in the month.

Dr. Judt, of Bremen University, was the first to use such a table; but after him engineer Hans Früh and other worked out several similar calculation charts. No matter what chart is used, however, the final resulting figures should be the same. Western charts involve calculating the first day of the given month. But calculations of the first day are not always valuable. This is especially true since, as I have mentioned, caution days are of primary importance in biorhythm, whereas plus and minus factors are merely of secondary significance.

I have evolved a simple calculating table for working out caution days for any given month and, to distinguish it from other similar devises, have called it the Tatai Simplified Direct Calculator. This device not only enables the beginner to calculate automatically the caution days of each cycle for any month, it also makes possible the development of the highly simplified *Biolucky* (see p. 69) scaling measurement system.

Using Quételet's law of distribution on a large number of cases, I found that this calculator is accurate in 70 percent of cases. In other words, it is not applicable to everyone. But a two- or three-year check of the degree to which it predicts caution days on which illness or other unfortunate occurrences happen shows that the system works well for large numbers of people. It is better to employ a system with a high degree of accuracy than to have no standard of judgment at all. A searchlight or an infrared light does not provide the illumination of full day, but it makes shooting at a target easier than it would be in complete darkness. Similarly this basic formula is more useful than none for the person just beginning to acquire and apply knowledge of biorhythm.

When biorhythm is used, not as a kind of fortune telling, but in conjunction with autogenic training and behavioral science, individual biological differences tend to be absorbed in average values. Application of total averages in connection with prevention of such things as accidents involving taxis tends to elevate the awareness of a need for safety and in this way to lower accident rates.

Direct Calculation of Caution Days

My method, a serious revision of the Judt-Früh's system, is a new way to calculate caution days directly. It incorporates tables A, B, and C (see pp. 139–153) and makes it possible to work out immediately the caution days for any given month. I have named the device used in this method the Tatai Simplified Direct Calculator and give examples of its use here for the reader's study.

At first, biorhythm was used to make caution days safe through prediction by calculation. The most important implication for the beginner is not plus or minus curves, but the prediction of caution days, those days when caution can prevent mishaps in connection with health and other aspects of daily life. Of course, fluctuations of the plus and minus curve are interesting as graphs. But there is no place in the true science of biorhythm for the semiastrological idea—often propounded by manufacturers of biorhythm gadgets and by insurance salesmen—that the plus phase is good and the minus phase bad. Biorhythmic science does claim, however, that skillful timing and balance in the use of the plus and minus phases is important.

The beginner must not expect to progress in the required skills too rapidly. First he must learn how to live carefully with his three caution days. Doing this and incorporating knowledge of one's own personal idiosyncracies and experiences take at least a year. Making skillful use of the plus and minus phases requires still another two years of assiduous study. Hurrying in this course of learning can only lead to disadvantage and error.

To serve the beginner in these efforts, the Japan Biorhythm Laboratory has devised a simplified direct calculator making it possible to calculate immediately the caution days in any given month. To prevent confusion with other similar calculating tables, this one has been given the name of its inventor: Tatai.

The following examples show how the calculating system is to be used.

Example One
Person A was born on December 1, 1938. The calculation shows his PSI caution days for December, 1973.

	P	S	I	
From Table A for 1938	12	27	1	(a)
From Table B, December 1	11	25	3	(b)
From Table C, December, 1973	+ 5	17	17	(c)
(a)+(b)+(c)	28	69	㉑	
(Subtract each number of cycle days so that the result is neither zero nor a negative number.)		−28		
	−23	−28		
	⑤	⑬		

The answer figures are enclosed in circles to prevent confusion. This example shows that the first caution days in the cycles are as follows: P—December 5, S—December 13, and I—December 21.

Example Two
Person B was born on March 1, 1928; this example shows his biorhythm conditions for March, 1974.

	P	S	I	
From Table A, 1928	17	15	12	(a)
(People born in leap years must be careful to use chart values for March to December for such years.)				
From Table B, March 1	12	2	25	(b)
From Table C, March, 1974	+ 7	11	26	(c)
(a)+(b)+(c)	36	㉘	63	
(Subtract each number of cycle days	−23		−33	
so that the results are neither zero nor				
a negative number.)	⑬		㉚	

The answer figures are enclosed in circles. This example shows that the first caution days in the cycles are as follows: P—March 13, S—March 28, and I—March 30. As explained in the bottom line of each of the examples, the days calculated are the first caution days in each cycle. For instance, in the P cycle, the midcycle days may be obtained by adding eleven to each of the first caution day. Adding twelve too gives another caution day, if the addition means that the resulting day falls within the total days of the month. Subtracting twelve from the number of the day in the Tatai calculator gives caution days again, if the resulting number falls within the month. For instance, in *Example one*, P is the fifth. Adding eleven gives the sixteenth, and adding twelve to this sum gives the twenty-eighth. Since it is impossible to subtract twelve from five without producing a negative number, the physical caution days for person A are December 5, 16, and 28. In the case of person B, in *Example two*, P is the thirteenth. Adding eleven gives the twenty-fourth. Subtracting twelve gives the first. Therefore the physical caution days for person B are March 1, 13, and 24.

The sensitivity caution days may be calculated on the basis of the same principle. For instance, adding or subtracting fourteen to or from the S day values gives the caution days if the result of the arithmetical operation falls within the number of days of the month. In *Example one*, the Tatai number for the sensitivity cycle is the thirteenth. Adding fourteen gives the twenty-seventh for the sensitivity caution day. In *Example two*, the Tatai number for S is the twenty-eighth. Subtracting fourteen from this gives the fourteenth for the midcycle sensitivity caution day.

For the intellectual cycle, the addition of sixteen to the initial caution day gives the midcycle caution day. Subtracting seventeen from the value in the results gives an intellectual caution day if the remainder falls in the number of days of the month. For instance, subtracting seventeen from twenty-one, the Tatai value for

Example one, gives four. This means that the fourth is an intellectual caution day. The Tatai intellectual caution day for *Example two* is the thirtieth; subtracting seventeen from it gives an intellectual caution day on the thirteenth. The development of the Tatai system, by means of which anyone can easily calculate his own caution days for all three cycles, is a great advance in the study of biorthythm. An important aim in its development was the desire to spare the beginner the complications often involved in older devices and enable him to make the required calculations readily and accurately. The device employed in these calculations is already manufactured under the name Biolucky (see p. 69). A simple dial that anyone can carry about easily, it has won the praises of people related to biorhythm studies all over the world as the best device of its kind.

When NBC television and others asked me why I had been able to prompt development in biorhythm study when such progress has been lacking in the West, where the field of endeavor originated, I made the following reply.

In the West, biorhythm is confused with astrology. From the very outset, Japanese studies have ignored mystical fatalism. We have followed the West in making analytical statistical studies of the tendency for accidents to occur on caution days. But it would be nonsense for us to repeat what has been done in the West in a desultory fashion and to make no more than a game of biorhythm.

I have felt it imperative to take the study out of the laboratory and to perform social experiments with it by using biorhythm to reduce traffic accidents. The enthusiasm for safety on the parts of several important train and transit companies in Japan has enabled me to do fruitful work in this field. The owners of taxi companies with whom I worked agreed that simply admonishing drivers to be careful and drive safely is insufficient and that autogenic training would produce better results. As an indication of my gratitude, at the 1972 conference of the Japanese Association for Biorhythm Research, as the president, I presented certificates of appreciation to the people who have cooperated with me in this campaign.

Biorhythm Calendar Tables

I shall now discuss the other way to determine PSI conditions for any day by means of a round dial called the Biocycle Mini and the specified A, B, and C biorhythm calendar tables. This method is the first of its kind to be developed in the course of biorhythm studies of my laboratory. I shall explain the system by using two examples.

Immediately Understanding PSI Conditions for a Given Day: Dr. Judt's tables are the oldest easy way to plot biorhythm; but, as I have said, they reveal only conditions for the first day of the given month. This means that some other method must be used to determine PSI conditions for the other days of the month. Biorhythm calendar tables are a new way devised to overcome this inconvenience. The easiest explanation of their use is examples.

Example One
Calculations of the PSI conditions for December 1, 1973, for person A, who was born on December 1, 1938.

	P	S	I	
From Table A for 1938	13	3	1	(a)
From Table B for December 1	11	2	29	(b)
From Table C for December, 1973	18	11	16	(c)
D is 1	+ 1	1	1	(d)
(a)+(b)+(c)+(d)	43	⑰	47	
(Subtract the numbers of the cycle days so that the result is neither zero nor a negative number.)	−23		−33	
	⑳		⑭	

The answer figures are enclosed in circles. As in the other calculating methods, the appropriate figures are taken from tables A, B, and C; and the numbers of days in each cycle are subtracted from the sums of these figures. The sole difference is the figure for D, the number of the day of the month for which the PSI conditions are required.

Example Two
Calculations of the PSI conditions for March 13, 1974 for person B, who was born on March 1, 1928.

	P	S	I	
From Table A for 1928	8	15	23	(a)
(Since the subject was born in March of a leap year, it is necessary to use March–December in the table.)				
From Table B for March 1	10	25	7	(b)
From Table C for March, 1974	16	17	7	(c)
D is 13	+13	13	13	(d)
(a)+(b)+(c)+(d)	47	70	50	
(Subtract the numbers of cycle days so that the result is neither zero nor a negative number.)	−23	−28		
	−23	−28	−33	
	①	⑭	⑰	

The answer figures are enclosed in circles. From *Example One*, the PSI conditions for person A on December 1, 1973, are as follows: P ⑳, S ⑰, and I ⑭. The Biocycle Mini, which I shall discuss next, gives this easy graphic representation. The pertinent figures in it show that the physical cycle is negative, the sensitivity cycle early negative, and the intellectual cycle late positive.

For *Example Two*, the PSI conditions for person B on March 13, 1974, are as follows: P ①, S ⑭, and I ⑰. From the Biocycle Mini, it becomes apparent that this person is experiencing a physical caution day; a sensitivity positive day, one day before caution day; and an intellectual caution day.

The Surprisingly Convenient Biocycle Mini: The basis of this method is the calculation of PSI conditions for a given day. It resembles other calculation methods in that it employs the sums of PSI numbers taken from tables A, B, and C of the biorhythm calendar. It differs from them, however, in calling for the addition to these sums of D, the number of the day for which the PSI conditions are needed. As was true in the other calculating method, the numbers of the days in each cycle must be subtracted (more than once if necessary to reach a minimum) from these sums without producing zero or a negative number. By referring the results of this operation to the Biocycle Mini, it is possible to tell the biorhythm conditions of the day at a glance. For instance, if the P number is one, the Biocycle Mini shows this figure in a red spade, indicating a physical caution day. If the P number is twelve, the day is also a caution day. If it is five, the person is in the physically positive phase; and if it is eighteen, he is about half way through the physically negative phase.

If the sensitivity number is fifteen, in the Biocycle Mini, it will be enclosed in a red heart; this means that the person must be careful about emotional changes. If the intellectual number is seventeen, it will be enclosed in a green club, indicating that this day may be one on which the person is forgetful. The Biocycle Mini is devised on standards set by the Japan Biorhythm Laboratory (JBL).

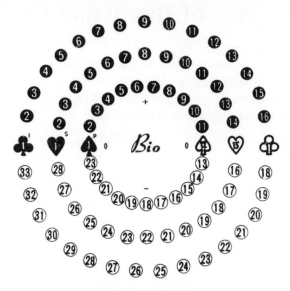

Biocycle Mini

The Biocycle Mini is surprisingly convenient in that it requires only printing and no rulers, as does another method that I shall explain. It will fit in address books or small pocket notebook. Ideally, it should be used in conjunction with biorhythm charts, biorhythm calendars, and small electronic eight-digit calculators. If physicians employ it in combination with calculators, the Biocycle Mini makes it possible to determine a patient's condition in about thirty seconds. The author's idea has been given electronic realization in the Casio-Biolator (see p. 70).

Correct Indication of Biorhythm Cycles

In this section, I discuss the Japan Biorhythm Laboratory (JBL) system of plotting biorhythm cycles. This system has been evolved by the JBL as most suitable in the light of our successful scientific work in traffic-accident reduction.

The numerous methods used to indicate biorhythm can be divided into three basic types: those that show only the given day, those that show the caution days, and those that show PSI conditions for one or two entire months, and in calendar fashion for as much as a full year. Problems related to all the types are manifested in the system that shows conditions for a month. In the following sections, I shall discuss the various indication systems.

Traditionally in Europe, the Früh system of a calendar arranged in columns read from top to bottom is used. The PSI conditions for the first day of the month are calculated by the Judt-Frueh simplified calculation tables. These PSI values are the basis on which the rest of the calendar is filled in. Recently, the columns of the calendars have been changed to horizontal lines to conform to the needs of the computers that are now widely used. The values for the first days of the month are fed to the computer, which automatically types in the conditions for the remaining days in the month. Though the major manufacturers of devices for this kind of indication system are in Germany and Switzerland, there are many in the United States and Japan as well.

In Japan, accurate scientific methods based on the standards of the Japan Biorhythm Laboratory are used to indicate biorhythm cycles under the following conditions.

(1) Blue is used for the physical cycle, red for the sensitivity cycle, and green for the intellectual cycle. Dr. Fliess determined that the physical cycle is masculine and the sensitivity cycle feminine. Just as in many folk customs, so in international scientific practice, blue is accepted as symbolic of the male and red of the female.

(2) When printing requirements forbid the use of colors, again in keeping with international scientific custom, the physical cycle is represented by solid lines, and the sensitivity cycle by broken lines. The intellectual cycle is represented by lines composed of dots and dashes.

(3) The Japan Biorhythm Laboratory does not regard caution days as evil. Instead it encourages positive autogenic training on such days, because, in this way, it is possible to limit accidents and unpleasant occurrences to which people are prone at these times. For this reason, we believe that, in biorhythm calendars, it is important to combine columns for conditions and others for personal memoranda. Unless these calendars are small, they cannot be carried about easily. They then lose much of their value for autogenic training. Furthermore, portability and ease of

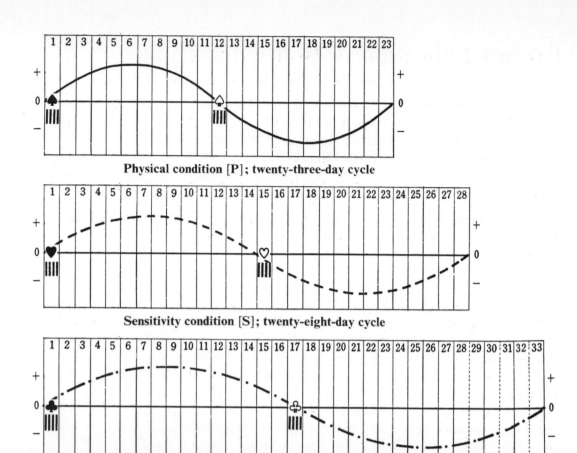

Physical condition [P]; twenty-three-day cycle

Sensitivity condition [S]; twenty-eight-day cycle

Intellectual condition [I]; thirty-three-day cycle

use are essential for the preparation of daily schedules and for jotting down episodes as they occur and compiling information for the analysis of pertinent personal idiosyncracies. To meet these needs, we have prepared monthly biorhythm calendars in which the column for a single day is four millimeters wide.

(4) The next thing required is a device making possible instantaneous recognition of biorhythm conditions. To meet this need, we have devised a transparent plastic scale. The three sides of the scale are curved to represent the physical, sensitivity, and intellectual cycles. Using it and a four-colored ballpoint pen, one can plot biorhythm conditions easily and accurately. It is essential to make marks on the plot indicating caution days, since these are the most important times in the cycles.

Because the positive and negative phases are of secondary importance and since the amplitude of fluctuation between them should be scientifically very small, our system has limited this amplitude to a minimum to prevent the individual from overemphasizing its ups and downs and mistakenly believing that positive is always good, negative always bad, and caution days always critical and disastrous.

To solve these problems, we limited the maximum amplitude to plus-minus ten millimeters. If the horizontal swing for one day is reduced to three millimeters, it would be a mistake from the standpoint of the correct representation of biorhythm

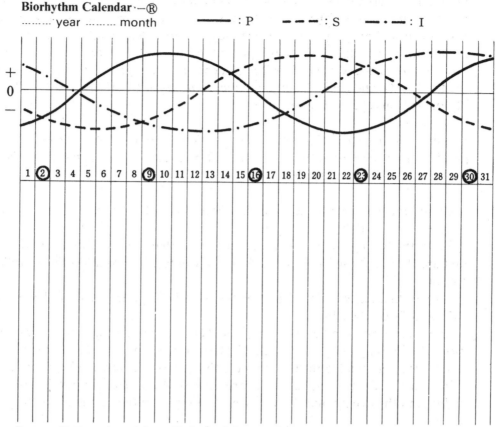

Biorhythm Calendar ·—®

········· year ········ month   ——— : P   --- : S   —·— : I

In this calendar, prepared for use with the autogenic training system, the memoranda column is large enough for extensive notations. The calendar is 14 centimeters by 12 centimeters. Each column is 4 millimeters wide.

not to reduce the amplitude accordingly to about seven millimeters.

(5)   Indication of the caution days must not be handled thoughtlessly. Dr. Fliess indicated a first cycle day as **XX** and a midcycle day as **X**. The JBL standards, which employ a fluctuation curve, do not need to indicate the caution days in such a way.

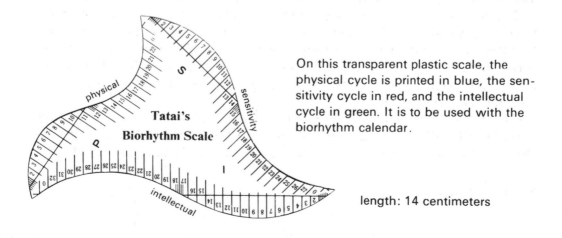

On this transparent plastic scale, the physical cycle is printed in blue, the sensitivity cycle in red, and the intellectual cycle in green. It is to be used with the biorhythm calendar.

length: 14 centimeters

We use four vertical lines to enable the person to make simple, yet accurate, ballpoint pen indications. The four lines show not only the first caution day, but also the midcycle day. This provides both accuracy and an orderly chart. To finish the chart according to JBL standards, Sundays are marked with red circles.

(6)   For instances in which ballpoint pens are not used, the JBL has introduced spades, hearts, and clubs. Even in monochrome representations, these symbols identify the various cycles at once.

Compiling a Biorhythm Calendar: This section is devoted to examples designed to provide practice in using the biorhythm calendar tables A, B, and C and the scale in preparing biorhythm calendars.

Example

Compiling a biorhythm calendar for December, 1973, for person A, who was born on December 1, 1938.

From the biorhythm calendar tables it is seen that the conditions for December first are P ⑳, S ⑰, and I ⑭. These figures are entered as explained in the following section.

(1)   With a black ballpoint pen, in the top column enter the dates December 1, 1938 and December, 1973.

(2)   Because December has thirty-one days, it is unnecessary in this case; but for months with only thirty days, use a black ballpoint to make a solid line on the dotted line between the thirtieth and the thirty-first to avoid confusion. The same thing must be done in the case of February with the dotted line between the twenty-eighth and the twenty-ninth or between the twenty-ninth and the thirtieth in leap years.

(3)   To plot the curve for the physical cycle, align the P ⑳ point of the scale with the first-day line of the calendar. Make sure that these lines are together throughout the entire space of the month. Next, carefully align the 0 line of the scale and the 0 line of the calendar. In drawing by scale, as anyone with drafting experience knows, the line produced may be in a slightly different position from the edge of the scale. To minimize this discrepancy, our scales are made of very thin plastic. The line produced by means of them is close enough to create no hindrance for practical purposes. Bringing the scale down a very small distance, however, will result in a still more accurate line.

(4)   Draw the physical-cycle line with blue ballpoint pen. In monochrome printed material, it is represented with a solid line. The scale is designed to draw only one cycle at a time. (Note that the cycles on the scale all end on zero and not on twenty-three, twenty-eight, and thirty-three.) When you have drawn the curve for one cycle, turn the scale so that the next cycle edge is uppermost and align it with the next pertinent day. Long scales, making possible the drawing of cycles for a full month without altering the scale's position are available for professionals who must draw large numbers of calendars.

(5)   When you have drawn the curve for the physical cycle throughout the month, align the IIII mark on the scale and draw four vertical lines as shown on p. 56. (The IIII is the caution-day mark.) These lines, of course, must be drawn with a blue

ballpoint pen.

(6)   Next align S ⑰ with the first day of the month on the calendar and draw the curve for the sensitivity cycle as explained in (3), (4), and (5) above. An example is shown in p. 57. Be sure to use a red ballpoint pen for this cycle. In monochrome printed matter, it will be shown with a broken line. Do not forget to make four marks for the caution day. A calendar that shows only the curves and omits the caution days cannot be called a scientific biorhythm calendar.

(7)   Follow the same procedure in drawing the curve for the intellectual cycle. Align I ⑭ with the first day of the month. Use a green ballpoint pen for both the line and the marks for the caution day. In monochrome printed matter, this line is composed of dots and dashes.

(8)   Make red circles around all of the Sundays in the month and red triangles around all the other holidays.

(9)   This concludes the compilation of a biorhythm calendar based on the scientific standards of the Japan Biorhythm Laboratory. If you wish to continue the calendar into the next month, it is unnecessary to calculate the succeeding PSI values. All you need to do is to align the PSI numbers following those for December 31 with January 1 and continue drawing curves. It is more efficient and less likely to lead to error if you draw first the physical-cycle line for as long as you wish. Then draw the other two curves, one at a time. Finally, put red circles around the Sundays and red triangles around the holidays. If you suspect errors in the drawing, check the biorhythm conditions of the last month you drew by calculating back from the biorhythm calendar tables. Then using the scale, check to see if the conditions expressed in the drawn calendar graph agree with the results of the calculations. If they do, the entire calendar graph is correct. It is still easier to make this check with the newly developed biorhythm electronic calculator Casio Biolator (see p. 70).

(10)   The calendar can be drawn with the help of the Tatai Simplified Direct Calculator, but one difference must be observed in plotting the curves. The Tatai table gives conditions for the initial caution day in the cycle. Consequently, to plot the curves, the ruler must be aligned on the initial caution day and not on the first day of the month.

For instance, in the first example given above, the initial physical critical day for the subject in the month of December is the fifth. In order to plot the physical-cycle curve, the first day of the physical-cycle side of the ruler must be aligned with the fifth of the month. The four blue vertical marks will be made on this day, and the plotted line will be drawn with a blue ballpoint pen. The line for the first four days of the month must be drawn by aligning them with the twentieth through the twenty-third with the scale.

(11)   The scale can be used in conjunction with the newly developed biorhythm electronic calculator—Casio Biolator—to plot curves for several months. If you press the key for the first day of the month for which information is needed, the calculator will provide the PSI conditions. These and the scale can be used to plot calendars for several months. Check the accuracy of the drawing by using the electronic calculator to work out the PSI conditions for the final month plotted and check the figures against the curves.

High-key and Low-key Phases

Having learned how to live successfully with caution days, you can increase the importance of biorhythm to the behavioral-scientific aspects of your life by paying attention to the way you live in the high-key and low-key phases of each cycle. In this section, I present basic, beginner-level information on this subject and on the topic of compatibility in its biorhythm sense.

There is a general tendency to regard the high-key, or positive, phase as good and the low-key, or negative, phase as bad. For people with no biological knowledge, this may be excusable. But it is an error and must be guarded against by persons who wish to make skillful application of biorhythm in their daily lives. I can give a very good reason for avoiding the idea that the high-key phase is necessarily good and can suggest why mistakes and trouble occur during it. People who tend to live ordinarily at a high-key (they are called hyperergic in biological terms) are like an automobile racing too fast down a highway. It is likely that they may meet disaster when they come to a sharp curve, since they will be going too fast to keep the car under control and will either crash into the guardrail or cross the centerline and run into oncoming traffic in the opposite lanes. Reckless people of this kind must regard the high-key phase of their cycles with the greatest caution of modesty.

To people who truly wish to make biorhythm the barometer of their daily life, it cannot be said too often that human beings are not mold-formed, mass-produced dolls. We all have flesh and blood; we are all different, not only because of our different hereditary compositions, but also because of the various past experiences that contribute to the creation of the people we are at present. Dr. Harold G. Wolff, the world-famous authority on psychosomatic medicine and the inventor of the Cornell Medical Index, put it well in his book *Stress and Disease*, when he said that physical makeup is the past experience of each individual. Biorhythm is a field of learning. It is an abstract matter. Therefore, to put it to use in daily life, you must begin by abandoning the mechanical assumption that high-key is good and low-key is bad.

For people who tend to live always in an excessively high-key, the low-key phase is an excellent time in which they can do their work smoothly and without mistake. In this and in many other aspects of life, what the Chinese call the Doctrine of the Mean is the best and safest policy. If moderation is not observed, illnesses of the heart and other serious sicknesses may develop.

To make good use of biorhythm in your daily life, you must take the test on p. 61 and employ the results to teach yourself how to make optimum application of your biorhythm calendar. The secret of success in this endeavor is to combine the test results, your biorhythm calendar, and your knowledge of your own personality:

Biorhythm Aptitude Check by JBL

P (Physical Cycle)	S (Sensitivity Cycle)	I (Intellectual Cycle)
+ { Prone to colds Prone to constipation Suffer from a weak liver Immediately speak ill of others Refuse to listen to advice Fond of oily foods	+ { Speak up often and readily in conferences Suffer from frequent headaches Have many friends Lose temper over small matters Careful about expenditures of money	+ { Have frequent bright ideas Worry often Easily disturbed by things Unhappy unless own ideas are pushed through Fond of pictures and handicrafts Fond of modern music
− { Prone to diarrhea Prone to fatigue Tend to be rheumatic Become thirsty easily Fond of light, simple foods Cannot fall asleep quickly at night	− { Sensitive to fashions Carefully put things away for preservation Suffer from stiff shoulders often Easily deceived by people Sentimental and romantic Physical condition perpetually poor Fond of cleanliness	− { Fond of mystery novels Plan things well Skillful at hand work Have good handwriting Enjoy listening to classical music Good marks in school

Encircle the characteristics in each cycle that pertain to you. If there is a difference of more than three between the plus and minus aspects encircled in each cycle or if there is a difference of more than five between the total plus and minus characteristics encircled, refer to the biorhythm aptitude advice found in the autogenic-training card (p. 62).

whether you are introverted or extroverted; whether you are negative or positive in general outlook.

In filling out the aptitude check, read the entire test twice, then make circles according to the instructions at the bottom of the page. Next refer to the autogenic-training card and use the information given there as reference in connection with your individual biorhythm calendar.

People for whom the amplitude of fluctuation between high-key and low-key phases is wide must take into consideration the question of compatibility for the sake of harmonious relations with others. Here I shall mention compatibility in terms

Biorhythm Autogenic-training Card by JBL

P (Physical Cycle)	S (Sensitivity Cycle)	I (Intellectual Cycle)
● If you have encircled more than six positive and negative elements, on zero caution days be wary of speeding, drinking, or any other activity that might upset you physically.	● If you have encircled more than six positive and negative characteristics, on zero caution days, be conservative; do not pass other cars if you are driving and do not be hasty to express your opinions.	● If you have encircled more than six positive and negative characteristics, on zero caution days, be especially careful to check stoplights before crossing streets and be cautious about losing things.
● If you have encircled more than three positive characteristics, be careful to do nothing rash or excessive during your positive phases.	● If you have encircled more than three positive characteristics, in your positive phases, be moderate in all things and respect the feelings of others.	● If you have encircled more than three positive characteristics, in your positive phases, do not be hasty or greedy; do your work carefully, piece by piece.
● If you have encircled more than three negative characteristics, be careful to rest adequately and to eat stamina foods during your negative phase.	● If you have encircled more than three negative characteristics, during your negative phases, strive to be positive and to avoid making unpleasantness for others.	● If you have encircled more than three negative characteristics, in your negative phases, get plenty of sleep and plan to do your work accurately in the mornings.

of a mathematical relationship. The meaning of *compatibility* in this case differs from the term as used in marital matters.

As I have said often, there are no absolute values in biorhythm. The dimensions of thought are different from considerations of mental or physical superiority. Bright and less bright people, strong and weak people all have good and bad days in terms of compatibility. Those differences become apparent if the variations occurring daily in their conditions are carefully examined. In other words, I am not discussing individual physical makeup or personality. In this case, compatibility is a way of categorizing people roughly on the basis of averages, overlooking subtle mood changes that take place each day, hour, and minute. The biorhythm aptitude check is one way of doing this. The biorhythm autogenic-training card is a systematized model way of planning the application of biorhythm to daily life and of finding out how to put autogenic training to most fruitful use. Because it invites misunderstanding, *compatibility rate* may not be the best term; but I intend to use it because I dislike the introduction of new, difficult terminology. It is essential to remember that biorhythm is dynamic and not static. Its very dynamic nature explains the difference between the word *compatibility* as used here and the same work in ordinary contexts.

To determine compatibility rate, let us think in terms of vectors as employed in dynamics. In connection with actual time, the word *scalar* is employed to express the direction, speed, volume, and force of a movement in a different direction from a given point—in three, four, or more dimensions. The following is an elementary explanation of compatibility rate employing vectors.

As an example, I shall take the sensitivity cycle of person A. Since the fourteenth day is the midpoint of this cycle, a person born on a day fourteen days before or after A's birthday has a sensitivity-cycle vector the opposite of A's. (The same would be true if the person were born forty-two, seventy, ninety-eight, or any number of days that is the sum of twenty-eight and its multiples plus fourteen days before or after A's birthday.) The compatibility rate of these two people is zero. If the difference between their days of birth is 7 or 21 days, their compatibility rate is 50 percent. This means that out of ten days, their high- and low-key phases coincide on five. Dividing 100 percent by 14 gives more than 7.14 percent of days on which they have a one-day gap. For biological purposes, it is sufficient to round this off to 7 percent. With this percentage, it is possible to plot a relationship graph like the one in the S zone of the chart below. Calculating in the same way for the physical and intellectual cycles produces a general biorhythm compatibility chart. The midpoints of the physical and intellectual cycles are 11.5 days and 16.5 days. The movement ratio of the days can be calculated by dividing 100 percent by these figures. Rounding off the results produces the compatibility ratios shown in the chart on p. 64.

But for biorhythm as a rule of living, such fine calculations are meaningless. It is enough to keep in mind the following general guide: compatibility of only 25 percent is not good, from 25 to 75 percent is good, and from 75 to 100 percent is excellent. Still people with different personalities, those whose compatibility rates are low, often tend to be on good terms. This statement is the outcome of consideration of experience with the sensitivity cycle. It is probably wise not to make generalizations about the physical and intellectual cycles.

Practically speaking, we can see the following differences in preferences and actions between people with low sensitivity-cycle compatibility rates. If A suggests a trip to a bowling alley or a hiking expedition, B, whose sensitivity cycle is incompatible with A's, will refuse, saying that she prefers to remain at home listening to records or reading. Two people whose personalities differ and who find it difficult to get along well together will learn, if they take the trouble to investigate, that their sensitivity-cycle compatibility ratios are low.

Twenty-eight-day sensitivity cycle

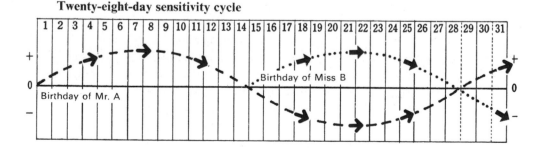

Compatibility Chart

Day Discrepancy	P	S	I
0	100	100	100
1	91	93	94
2	83	86	88
3	74	79	82
4	65	71	76
5	57	64	70
6	48	57	64
7	39	50	58
8	30	43	52
9	22	36	46
10	13	29	39
11	4	21	33
12	4	14	27
13	13	7	21
14	22	0	15
15	30	7	9
16	39	14	3
17	48	21	3
18	57	29	9
19	65	36	15
20	74	43	21
21	83	50	27
22	91	57	33
23	100	64	39
24		71	46
25		79	52
26		86	58
27		93	64
28		100	70
29			76
30			82
31			88
32			94
33			100

Importance of the Law of Initial Value

I have already explained that there are no absolute values in biorhythm, which consists of wave motions in the gentle and minute fluctuations in the mind and body. It is because of their very minuteness, that it is difficult to conduct on them the kind of clear scientific study that has been performed on circadian cycles. Nonetheless, the American scholar Dr. Joseph Wilder has formulated the law of initial value, which is of great importance to biorhythm.

Dr. Joseph Wilder, of New York University, first formulated the law of initial value (LIV) in about 1930. It involves basimetry (*Ausgangswertgesetz*), or the measurement of basal values, and is of vital importance to the realistic aspects of biological rhythms.

If the first pulse beat is strong, no matter what the biorhythm phase, the pulse rate will remain strong; that is, it will continue to beat at a high level. A child who is hereditarily intelligent, even in his low-key phases, is brighter than a child who is unintelligent, even when the latter is in his high-key phases. Similarly, a person who is physically strong, even in his low-key phases, is more than a match for a weak man at his best. For instance, no matter that he is in his high-key phase, the rank amateur cannot hope to win a boxing match with a professional. The law of initial value provides another good reason for diligence in training in daily life.

Of course, there are individual differences among the amplitudes or grades of fluctuation in the physical, sensitivity, and intellectual wave phenomena. My studies have shown that women tend to manifest greater emotional fluctuation than men. But some people, regardless of sex, are governed by emotions to a larger extent than others.

After having made calculations and compiled biorhythm calendars, many people easily fall into the delusion that the positive phase is good and the negative phase bad. Particularly people who have no background in biology make this mistake. It is clearly audacity for a person to claim to be a specialist merely because he teaches others how to plot biorhythm calendars on a level with kindergarten learning. It is only that, by coincidence, some people have learned how to draw the calendars early and can teach what they know to others. No matter how many times I repeat this, it cannot be overemphasized. If there is someone in your acquaintance who pretends to be a teacher and who insists that the positive phase is good and the negative phase is bad, under no circumstances believe him. The biological living system is healthy only when positive and negative phases are well balanced. But I shall leave this topic for more detailed discussion later.

Another important contribution of the law of initial value to the study of bio-rhythm can be illustrated by the following example. A doctor, believing that medicine

A will cure a given sickness with effect α, prescribes it for his patient. If, instead of the desired effect α, effect β is produced, the doctor may call β a side-effect. Sometimes, medicine A may take effect but produce only about half of the desired result. In certain instances, the medicine even has an adverse effect. This is especially true in cases of treating upsets in the nervous and endocrine systems, as the biorhythm authority Professor Arne Sollberger says. My more than thirty years of study on these topics convince me that he is correct.

Experience with work on responses in the autonomic nervous system first brought the need for the establishment of something like the law of initial value to the attention of Dr. Wilder. At present, psychologists are very interested in the law. In mental sicknesses, what is called the crisis and paradoxical responses often occur. For instance, the smoker turns to cigarettes for relief from tension in the para-sympathetic nervous system when he is tired and in a low-key state. The same smoker turns to cigarettes again for relief from tension in the sympathetic nervous system when he is excited and irritable. There are instances in which the same volume of a medicine to reduce blood pressure lowers the blood pressure of a high-blood-pressure patient, has no effect on a normal patient, and raises the blood pressure of a low-blood-pressure patient. These brilliant illustrations are taken from the work of Dr. Arne Sollberger.

From the standpoint of the law of initial value, it is understandable that stimulation to a person in a high-key state produces little effect, whereas depression produces a great one. Conversely, stimulation to a person in a low-key phase produces a great effect, whereas depression produces a small one. A doctor who thoroughly understands the roles of the sympathetic and parasympathetic systems within the autonomic nervous system would not find the case of the smoker and his paradoxical responses to nicotine unusual.

The graph on p. 67 shows a biorhythm cycle—both high- and low-key phases— in relation to this phenomenon. Though it manifests itself in all three cycles, it is easiest to understand in the emotional cycle. As the chart shows, there is a fixed limit to the high-key phase; it cannot be expanded indefinitely. When the stimulus from without is great, biological energy reaches the limit and must be compressed. When the energy passes its limits it produces distortions in the form of stress in the body. Knowledge of the law of initial value makes it easy to understand why high-key daily living produces prolonged stress. Autogenic training is useful in relieving this stress. Indeed it is probably more effective in dealing with high-key than with low-key conditions. The physical and personal differences among the high-key limits of various people show how nonsensical it is to assume that high-key is always good.

The relationships in the low-key phase are the same, except that fewer natural stimuli tend to lower the key further. Of course, it is necessary to be wary of tran-quilizers and sleeping pills. Natural stimuli in such cases provide even better recovery than in the high-key phase, as the chart clearly shows. Stimuli that exceed the limit, however, lead to chronic fatigue and lack of sleep and can in this way become the cause of a slump condition. The many people who complain of slump in their biorhythm negative phases are probably ignoring the law of initial value. The negative phase, if used correctly, is in no way inferior to the positive. Actually in

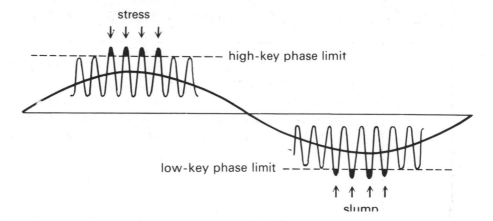

stress

high-key phase limit

low-key phase limit

slump

Relations between high-and low-key phases

hyperergic persons, high-key is apt to be associated with crimes of violence. Actual examples will be illustrated later.

The Biolucky Disk and Other Systems

The Tatai Biolucky disk is the most convenient device of its kind in the world. In this chapter, I explain how to use it. I add explanations of new biorhythm wristmeters, miniature calculators, and the computer panel board developed by the Japan Biorhythm Laboratory for use in safety control of groups of as many as thirty people.

Biolucky Dial: The Biolucky dial-type disk enables you to determine caution days at a glance. It is composed of one thick white plastic circular disk and three, thinner transparent plastic disks. On the white disk is a row of numbers in black circles. These numbers are the days of the calendar months and the PSI values from the Tatai charts. The numbers to thirty-one are in white against black for the sake of easy legibility. In addition, there are the numbers thirty-two and thirty-three, which are needed for calculating conditions in the intellectual cycle. The first of the inner transparent disks represents the physical cycle. It has a solid blue spade on its tab. Turning the disk by means of this tab, align the physical-cycle value calculated from the Tatai charts with the appropriate calendar day. This enables you to tell the physical-cycle condition for an entire month at a glance. Spades indicating the caution days are outline figures. Solid circles indicate days in the positive phase; outline circles indicate days in the negative phase.

It is an error to attempt to be mathematically completely correct in calculating caution days, especially those in the middle of the phase. For instance, in the case of the physical cycle, a male factor, which is twenty-three days, the middle caution day falls during the twenty-four hours between the afternoon of the twelfth and the morning of the thirteenth. But from the biological standpoint, it is wrong to disregard entirely the other twelve hours in each of the days. Although it is possible to think that, during these hours, conditions are less meaningful than during the twenty-four hours of the caution day, they deserve attention nonetheless. The individual differences in the accuracy of knowledge about the hour of birth further reveal the impossibility of adhering only to calendar dates in caution-day calculations. This and the fact that births tend to be more numerous in the morning hours led us to make the twelfth the caution day of the physical cycle in the Tatai dial and to eliminate consideration of the thirteenth. Furthermore, we believe this is correct since divergences to earlier days are more common than divergences to later days.

Taking the example given in the preceding chapter, align the physical-cycle dial tab with the fifth. This shows that throughout the month, other caution days occur on the sixteenth and the twenty-eighth. The days from the sixth through the fifteenth and those from the twenty-ninth through the thirty-first constitute the positive phase. The remaining days are the negative phase.

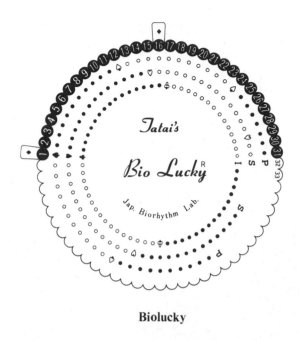

Biolucky

The tab for the sensitivity cycle is marked with a suitably feminine red heart. Once again, follow the example given in the preceding section and align the red-heart tab with the thirteenth. This shows at once that the thirteenth and twenty-seventh are caution days, that the days between the fourteenth and the twenty-sixth are the positive phase, and that the remaining days of the month are the negative phase.

The innermost disk, marked with green clubs, indicates the intellectual cycle. On the basis of the example in the preceding chapter, align the green-club tab with the twenty-first. It immediately becomes apparent that the fourth and the twenty-first are the caution days. The period between the first and the third and the period between the twenty-second and the thirty-first are marked with solid circles, indicating the positive phase.

The edges of the disks are scalloped to assist you in aligning them accurately. It is possible to attach the dial to walls or desks in a variety of ways. A tack may be driven through the hole in the center. A small magnet may be used to attach the disk to metal surfaces, or tape or other adhesives may be applied to the rear of the white **disk.**

Individual Biorhythm Wristmeters: In order to be of any value in the representation of the unbroken flow of biorhythm, a meter must not be allowed to run down, for if it does, adjustments are difficult to make. Of course, electric wall-clock-style meters involve less likelihood of this, but they are usually designed for use by large numbers of people and are therefore meaningless for the representation of anything as intensely individual as biorhythm conditions. The recent development of electronic wristwatches that run for as much as a year on a small battery has made possible the invention of a wristmeter for biorhythm. But, since all adjustments of such meters must be made by professionals and since the devices are strictly individual in

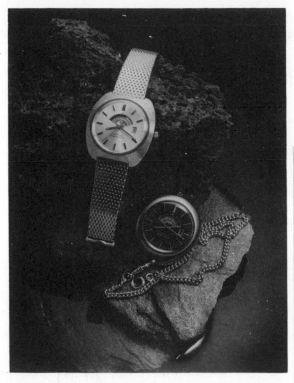

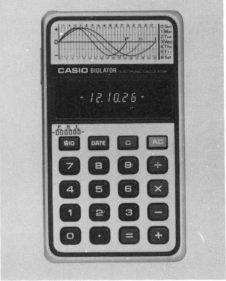

application, so far, they remain luxuries for the person who has intense interest in the field.

The World's First Pocket Biorhythm Calculator: The first pocket digital biorhythm calculator in the world has a special electronic brain capable of working out all time periods with a few operations of the keys. A touch of the BIO key converts this information into the three biorhythm stages, indicated by code numbers on the display. It can give any day in the years from 1901 to 1999. Automatic adjustments are made for leap years. It is small enough to be carried in the pocket.

Convenient Safety-control and Group-use Panel: A memory-device specialist conditioner panel has been developed to show at a glance the PSI conditions for thirty or more persons. It is especially useful for companies, for supervisors responsible for numbers of people, and for schools.

All the kinds of systems I have discussed—Judt's, the Tatai system, and others—share one important principle. They all involve individual differences because they all employ charts A and B, which are based on the date of birth (Biorhythm Calendar Table A and B). Chart C, on the other hand, is unrelated to individual conditions (Tatai Table C). This chart depends on the date of the day for which information is desired. The principle was analyzed and applied to make the group-use panel system.

1.   The value obtained by calculating the individual's date of birth on the A and B charts is a code number for any given person's PSI conditions. It does not change throughout a lifetime.

2.   In the group-panel system of representation, the code number is replaced with the actual name of the person in question, and the name is entered on the card corresponding to the numbers of days in the particular cycle. The three cards for PSI are arranged on a single panel and moved from day to day, enabling the supervisor or teacher to see all individuals' biorhythm conditions at a glance.

3.   The three PSI name cards become memory-device computers enabling the supervisor to check the conditions of the entire group. The device, called Biocondi-tioner, is shown below.

The panel is made of a piece of cardboard 22 by 29 centimeters and 2.5 centimeters thick. Of course, it can be used at the desk; but it is light and small enough to be carried in a briefcase.

The actual use of the panel is as follows. Let us assume that the panel is for a class of thirty students. First, it is necessary to prepare a list showing the dates of birth of all the students. Next, prepare a list of the P, S, and I values for each student, using the A and B charts. Values for the physical cycle must fall between one and

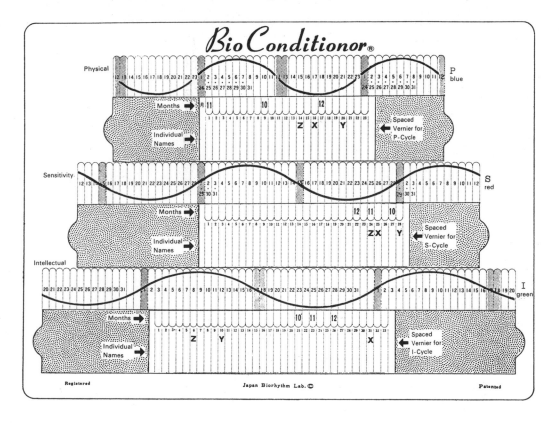

twenty-three, those for the sensitivity cycle between one and twenty-eight, and those for the intellectual cycle between one and thirty-three. If the sum worked out from two tables is greater than these numbers, subtract the number of days in the given cycle from it. Enter the name of each student in the columns corresponding to his P, S, and I values. Use a pencil so that the entries can be erased later, if necessary. It will not be surprising if more than one name is entered in a given column or if there are columns without names. Next, using chart C, find out the value of the month in question and enter the number in the appropriate column. Use a pencil and erase entries for the previous month so that the chart will always be up-to-date. The actual name cards can be moved. The number of the month (for instance, twelve for December) and the number of the day (for example, ten) will be combined. Sliding the cards from day to day will give the PSI conditions of the entire group at a glance. The sample panel makes it possible to see the daily PSI conditions of any group of about thirty people.

Caution for Beginners

Biorhythm is a science: the biological study of human cycles. Consequently, only people with specialized knowledge of medicine and biology are qualified to teach biorhythm properly. All other people tend to distort it. Of course, in medicine, as in all other things, there are grades of knowledge; and the beginner can understand in his own way. But, if mistaken things are learned at early stages in the course of education, they are extremely difficult to correct at later stages. If you have any mistaken information or ideas about biorhythm, it is important to correct them as quickly as possible. To aid you in doing this, I shall now discuss five points on which beginners require special caution.

1. *Marking Caution Days Accurately:* It is of the greatest importance always to mark the caution days accurately on your biorhythm calendars. Indeed, a calendar that is inaccurately or carelessly marked is virtually worthless. There are many ways of marking the caution days, though not all of them are as good as others. Engineer Früh used X marks. Some manufacturers or computerized calendars use the letter K or a circle. The Japan Biorhythm Laboratory uses two systems.

In one system, four vertical lines (IIII) mark the caution days. One set of four lines for the physical cycle is made in blue ballpoint pen; another set for the sensitivity cycle is made in red ballpoint pen; and a third set of four is made for the intellectual cycle in green ballpoint pen. These sets of four lines make it possible to display precisely not only the initial caution days in a cycle, but the midcycle caution days as well, even when, as in the case of the physical and intellectual cycles, the caution twenty-four hours straddle two calendar days.

A second system used by the Japan Biorhythm Laboratory has been devised for monochrome printed material. In such cases, the physical caution days are marked with spades, the sensitivity caution days with hearts, and the intellectual caution days with clubs. When possible, as in the Biolucky dial, the spade is blue, the heart red, and the club green. These biorhythm colors correspond to internationally understood biological color symbols: blue for masculinity and red for femininity. The physical cycle is considered masculine, and the sensitivity cycle feminine. Indeed, in some European countries, the physical cycle is designated M for man and the sensitivity cycle W for woman.

2. *Correct Indication of the Cycle Curves:* The only acceptable way to represent biorhythm cycle curves on calendars is the one advocated by the Japan Biorhythm Laboratory: solid line for the physical cycle, broken line for the sensitivity cycle, and a line composed of dots and dashes for the intellectual cycle.

3. *Correct Representation of the Positive and Negative Phases:* To counter the decidedly false notion that the positive phase is all **good** and the negative phase

all bad—a mistaken idea that I cannot refute often enough—it is important to limit representation of the positive and negative phases of each cycle to no more than a simple + or − or the high and low signs advocated by the Japan Biorhythm Laboratory. Under no circumstances should peak and valley indicators be used, as these suggest that positive is good and negative bad, when the truth is that human beings are able to live healthy lives only when balance is maintained between these two phases.

4. *Correct Attitude toward Caution Days:* Do not feel that caution days are necessarily times in which something bad is bound to happen. Do not be afraid of them. We all have good days and bad days. We are not machines and are sometimes healthy and sometimes prone to sickness. If we know the days on which we are in danger of illness or unpleasantness, we can take measures to protect ourselves. If a person goes out without knowing of the likelihood of rain, he can get wet and catch cold, or he can skid on wet pavement if he is driving. If that same person knows it is going to rain, he can wear a raincoat, drive with extra care, or stay home to protect himself from loss or danger.

I recommend that the beginner regard caution days as times in which to lead a normal, but careful, life. This is greatly assisted by proficiency in autogenic training. It is unwise, however, to undertake anything new on such days because this causes stresses that may lead to trouble. Use the caution days as times to develop powers of thought.

Days that are caution days in two or three of your cycles will occur, at most, once in a month. In the early stages of your study of biorhythm, live those days more cautiously but in an ordinary fashion. In this way you will get safely through the unstable times.

5. *Correct Understanding that Biorhythm is Not Fortune-telling:* Since biorhythm is a biological law, the plots we make for them are not 100 percent accurate. If they were, they would be a highly reliable kind of fortune-telling. Our interpretations of biorhythm cycles are accurate to only about 70 percent. My study of accidents occurring on the Japanese National Railways indicate that mishaps tend to center on the caution days with a slight tendency to deviation to the day before. Something similar is true of individual cases. Averages show that about 15.4 percent of all people tend to experience actual caution days on the day before the plotted caution day, whereas only 5.3 percent experience actual caution days the day after the plotted one. For this reason, the day before the plotted caution day is called the semicaution day to indicate that it deserves attention. Of course, consideration must be taken of the fact that the semicaution days preceding the midcycle caution days of the physical and intellectual cycles straddle two calendar days.

It would be of dubious value, however, to introduce semicaution days carelessly into statistical studies, where absolute accuracy is important. As the number of caution and semicaution days increase, the numbers of accidents and deaths occurring on them increase. This alters the balance of frequency and therefore causes changes in the methods of handling the statistics. A biorhythm study that fails to take this balance into consideration is unscientific.

Part 3

Practical
Examples and
Implications

Preventing Air Accidents

Flying an airplane demands great technical skill and is likely to involve unusual stresses. In the following section, I analyze biorhythm-related aspects of aircraft accidents that have occurred in Japan and refer to research material on the subject from other countries in an attempt to emphasize points demanding caution and attention.

In July, 1971, three horrible air accidents occurred in Japan. On the third, a domestic YS11, called Bandai, with sixty-eight people on board, crashed. On the sixteenth, a Self-defense Forces antisubmarine plane with eleven people on board crashed. And, on the thirtieth, a domestic Boeing 727 liner, with 162 people on board, collided in midair with a Self-defense Forces F86F jet fighter. The number of lives lost in these disasters was 241. In addition the costs in material damage, grief, and loss of morale were immense. Examination of the biorhythm calendars of the pilots involved in the tragedies reveals some highly important things.

Bandai: The crash of this YS11 took place on the afternoon of July 3, 1971.
It turned out that the pilot, named Terada, was experiencing a caution day in his intellectual cycle at the time. The copilot, an American named Spence, was experiencing a physical caution day. Furthermore, the previous day had been his intellectual caution day.

A year later, an investigation panel decided that the plane had crashed into a mountainside, which, because of fog, the pilot mistakenly judged to be Hakodate Airport. Why should he have made such a wild misjudgement? Conditions at the airport were not severe enough to interfere with landing. Indeed, planes before and after this one had all landed safely. No malfunction in the plane was discovered. The only explanation seems to be a mistake on the part of the pilot.

From the biorhythm standpoint, the most disturbing factor is the intellectual-cycle caution day of the pilot, especially in the light of the fact that he was instructing copilot Spence. As I shall explain in greater detail later, a crash of this kind is never the result of a single factor. It occurs as the consequence of an evil cycle of causes. Nonetheless, the intellectual caution day of the pilot, who was already in the uncomfortable position of having to instruct his copilot in a foreign language, causes concern and stress. Perhaps the tragedy could have been avoided if the caution days of the two men had been reversed; that is, if the pilot had been in a physical and the copilot in an intellectual caution day.

Self-defense Forces Jet Fighter: This accident took place early in the morning on the sixteenth of July. The pilot, a captain named Shimanuki, was a veteran. He was flying in his own home territory. For some reason, a wing tank caught on a pine

Biorhythm conditions of the people connected with several air accidents on the days on which the accidents occurred

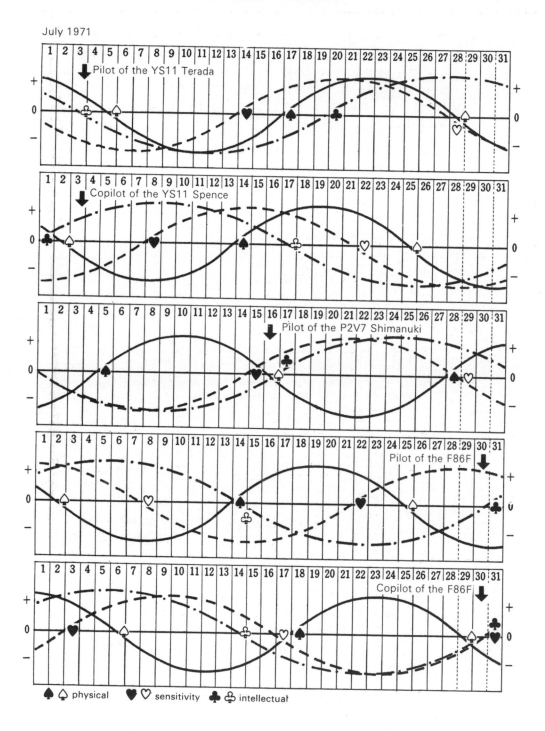

July 1971

♠ ♤ physical   ♥ ♡ sensitivity   ♣ ♧ intellectual

tree at the edge of the runway as he was about to land and fell off. Control tower told him to circle and make another landing try. He then disappeared over the waters of a nearby bay. The causes of the accident remain a mystery, though it is known that the pilot was in ominous biorhythm conditions: the day was an overlapping of caution days in all three cycles.

Collision between a Jet Liner and a Fighter: This accident was especially shocking because it occurred in broad daylight on a day when the weather was clear and apparently ideal for air travel. When I heard of the collision, I felt a cold chill up my spine. Since attending lectures by the famous specialist in the human element in automobile and aircraft accidents Dr. Ross A. McFarland, at Harvard, twenty years ago, I have been accustomed to refuse to take planes that arrive in the evening, no matter how busy I am, because statistics show that mistakes in landings by commercial flights are most common at that time of day. Conceivably Dr. McFarland and I, following the statistics, might have been perfectly content to board that plane, since it was traveling in bright daylight.

Investigation showed that the biorhythm conditions of the pilot and copilot of the commercial liner were good. Those of the pilot and copilot of the Self-defense Forces jet were bad and were similar to those of the pilot and copilot of the Bandai. The pilot was in a semicaution day in his intellectual cycle and was caught in a condition in which his sensitivity cycle was in the positive and his physical cycle in the negative phase. The copilot, who had only sixteen hours of training time, was in the same unfortunate condition as Shimanuki: the day of the accident was one in which caution days in all three of his cycles overlapped. In short, the instructor-pilot was in a bad biorhythm condition for the work he was called on to do; and the trainee-copilot was highly inexperienced.

Biorhythm Assisting in an Emergency: Of course, I do not intend to imply that biorhythm conditions are the only important factor in accidents. There is no assurance that catastrophes in the air will not occur as long as biorhythm conditions of the pilot are good. On the other hand, data is available to show that good biorhythm conditions can help people meet danger with the needed composure.

On the evening of July 19, 1971, a Japan Airlines DC8 jet liner took off from Tokyo International Airport on a flight to Hokkaido. Shortly after takeoff, an electrical storm caused hail, which struck against the aircraft and damaged the radar cone on the nose. The plane was flying a preset course, but the windshield glass in front of the copilot's seat was broken, as was the copilot's speedometer. The pilot, whose name was Stanton, immediately requested and got permission for an emergency landing. Fortunately, nearby was a consort plane. Stanton requested it to fly parallel so that he could check the accuracy of his own speedometer. Before long, the plane made a safe emergency landing at Tokyo International.

Investigation showed that, on the day, Stanton was in the positive phase of his physical and intellectual cycles and the negative phase of his sensitivity cycle. These were ideal biorhythm conditions for dealing with sudden accidents. Combined with the skill and experience of the pilot, they made possible a completely safe landing.

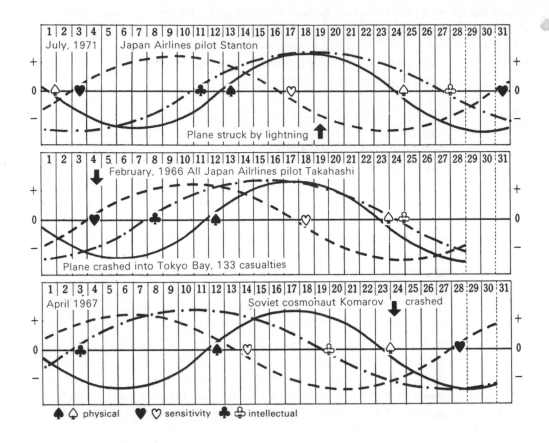

| 1 | 2 | 3 | 4 | 5 | 6 | 7 | 8 | 9 | 10 | 11 | 12 | 13 | 14 | 15 | 16 | 17 | 18 | 19 | 20 | 21 | 22 | 23 | 24 | 25 | 26 | 27 | 28 | 29 | 30 | 31 |

July, 1971   Japan Airlines pilot Stanton

Plane struck by lightning

February, 1966 All Japan Airlines pilot Takahashi

Plane crashed into Tokyo Bay, 133 casualties

April 1967   Soviet cosmonaut Komarov   crashed

♠ ♤ physical   ♥ ♡ sensitivity   ♣ ♧ intellectual

Crash of an Aerosbal: In January, 1973, an aerosbal, gathering information over the Pacific Ocean on a lost ship, was caught in a reverse wind. The pilot forgot about conserving enough fuel for the return trip. On the way home, they ran out of fuel; and the craft plunged into the ocean, taking the lives of three people. This accident was clearly the result of the mistake of the pilot, who was at the time experiencing a sensitivity caution day and a physical semicaution day.

A few days after the tragedy, a friend of the pilot called on me. A businessman and an amateur pilot, he brought a set of statistics compiled by him over more than a decade. His work showed that, in 121 air crashes in the Self-defense Forces, and commercial lines in Japan, twice as many occurred on pilot caution days as on noncaution days. The Zürich Airport Bureau allegedly made a study that showed that over one-third of sixty air crashes occurred on pilot caution days.

But watching biorhythm conditions alone is not enough to reduce the numbers of air accidents, which result from a conflux of causes, each of which must be studied and dealt with. I have found that the following things are true about air accidents. (1) Mistakes in landing occur often at airports located near the sea, lakes, deserts, or grassy plains. (2) Jet overshooting is a frequent cause of accidents. (3) Mistakes occur often in landings attempted in the evening and night. Elements (1) and (3) involve human physiological factors; (2) is connected with the physical performance of the aircraft. If we add biorhythm conditions as (4) to this set, we can make some pertinent remarks about the probabilities of accidents. For the sake of clarity, let us assign a value of thirty to each of these four elements and say that accidents do not occur unless the total of these elements amounts to more than one hundred. This means that even if elements (1), (2), and (3) are present or even if elements (2), (3), and (4) are present, accidents probably will not occur, for in both cases, the total value is only ninety. If all four are present, however, the likelihood is that an accident will take place. As a health designer, I propose the following system for the reduction of air accidents.

1. Make maximum efforts for health control. The close relation between the physical and mental states of the human entity means that, if a person suffers from a bad stomach or intestinal trouble, his abilities as a driver decrease. A pilot, who is often responsible for a large number of lives, must make certain that he remains in the best physical health in order that he may do his work with maximum mental alertness.

On February 14, 1968, the veteran Soviet cosmonaut Komarov, aboard Soyuz I, sent word to earth that further flight would be difficult and requested permission to return. He started a descent, but crashed upon landing. No one knows why he did not employ the emergency escape equipment. Furthermore, the reasons for his decision to curtail his voyage are uncertain. Did he have a heart attack? Was there a malfunction in the spacecraft? Komarov was a man of great skill and experience. An investigation of his biorhythm chart shows that his physical cycle was at its worst caution day and that both his sensitivity and intellectual cycles were in negative phases.

2. Carry out an autogenic training program enabling the pilot to overcome his personal faults and to act with maximum speed and efficiency. As long as the weather is good and the machine operates as it should, piloting an aircraft is easier than driving a car. The pilot can even sleep if he likes. But when weather changes or malfunctions develop, as they are apt to do without warning, the danger is immense, especially if there are many people on board. Under such conditions, the pilot must exert Promethean efforts to solve the problems facing him. The explosion of the Apollo XII dramatically illustrates the way in which mechanical failures can cause disaster. But often, there is a way to safety; and it is the pilot's heavy responsibility to exert maximum effort and skill to find it.

3. Use biorhythm calendars in planning pilots' work schedules. Pilots have more free days than drivers of ground vehicles. It is imperative to plan their work schedules so that two or three overlapping caution days do not fall on duty days. This will enable pilots to be prepared physically and mentally to meet whatever emergencies may arise.

4. Pilots should not be called on to instruct on caution days in their intellectual cycles. (This is true of such personnel as instructors in driving schools as well. Scheduling them so that they do not instruct on intellectual caution days reduces both accidents and the amounts of money that must be spent on repairs.)

As a specialist in biorhythm, I can say that, at present, not only flight hours and numbers of landing and takeoffs, but also the human elements as emphasized by Dr. McFarland, are being regarded too lightly and that this contributes to the large number of serious air accidents that occur. There are many such human elements, for instance, home life. I feel that it is wrong to make pilots fly international flights, which involve time lag, during the period beginning at the wife's sixth month of pregnancy and lasting through the first six months after birth. An airline that employs a large number of young pilots is running grave danger if it overlooks such elements and the pilots' biorhythm conditions. The magazine *International Aviation* published a report to the effect that, of 300 accidents involving English aircraft in a single year, 70 percent were traceable to mistakes in human operations or supervision. More than half were traceable to fatigue on the part of the pilots; in some cases, the pilots dozed while on duty. It seems that the biorhythm of the pilot of the Japan Airlines plane that crashed in Moscow, on November 29, 1972, was inauspicious.

H.W. Heinrich, of Travelers Insurance Company, U.S.A., a specialist in the study of accidents, said that, for every accident that actually occurs, there are twenty-nine latent ones and three hundred minor causes of trouble. Any one of these could be the trigger that, if pulled, could start an avalanche of disaster. For this reason, I cannot insist too strongly that airlines and people related to this kind of travel devote maximum attention to the human elements and the biorhythm conditions that are intimately connected with causes of accidents.

The Swiss pilot Werner Tschannen analyzed 513 aircraft accidents and learned that 377 of them (73.5 percent) are related to poor biorhythm conditions (caution first days and midcycle days or negative phases in two or more cycles). Details of his work will appear in *Biorhythm in the World Today*, to be published in 1978. In research on 270 accidents involving military aircraft, he learned that 1.75 times as many occur on pilot physical caution days as on pilot noncaution days.

Studies of 110 accidents involving Japanese Self-defense Force aircraft between 1955 and 1974 reveal that 1.44 times as many take place on pilot physical caution days and 1.47 times as many on pilot sensitivity caution days as on noncaution days. Differences related to positive and negative phases appeared only in the case of the intellectual cycle, in which 1.58 times as many accidents occurred on caution as on noncaution days.

Since the number of cases was small, these findings remain largely provisional. They are nonetheless interesting because they show that, both in Japan and Switzerland, pilots of military craft, in which safety is sometimes sacrificed to performance, tend to be strongly influenced by physical conditions.

I have heard that some American airlines give new pilots biorhythm calendars. This is certainly a good idea and a contribution to the safety strategy. Still more valuable is the suggestion that Dr. Douglas E. Neil, of the Naval Postgraduate School, and Dr. Stuart O. Persons, of the Lockheed Aircraft Corporation, made at the International Air Transport Association twentieth technical conference, in November, 1975, to the effect that the use of biorhythm ought to go beyond personal application by individual pilots and ought to be put to practical use in scheduling work and improving personnel relations.

Reduction of Traffic Accidents

In the hope of reducing the large number of traffic accidents occurring in Japan, in 1967, I instituted a biorhythm program that was soon adopted by transit companies and many other organizations, with the result that, in a short while, accidents were lowered by as much as from one-third to three-fourths. At present, the program is employed by electrical power companies throughout the nation and by the Japan Self-defense Forces. In the following section, I outline the major points of this program.

The automobile has become so important a part of modern civilization that some specialists are now saying that, in the employment of it and of other machines, human beings are rapidly depleting the amounts of usable energy on the planet and may be unable to survive another century. Certainly one of the most automobile-minded people on earth is the Americans, by whom the family car is regarded as a necessity. In cities like New York, which have more or less well-developed public transportation systems, some people have given up the family car. For instance, a medical practitioner whom I first met at a conference in Vienna and who lives in New York told me that he had sold his car because parking was difficult and traffic was dangerous. He feels that buses, taxis, and the subway systems provide all the transportation he needs. Other Americans, on the other hand, cannot give up their cars if they are to continue to live in the much-admired suburban areas and commute to cities to work, because the American train system is no longer satisfactory. Often commuting takes over an hour, but the Americans solve the problem of distance and expense by organizing car pools. A number of people living in the same suburban or rural region and working in the same city form a group. On a rotational basis, each member of the group drives the other members to work for a day or a set number of days. If the distance is great, the members of the pool relieve each other at the steering wheel so that no one becomes exhausted from driving. If the Japanese would adopt a similar system, they would reduce pollution caused by automobiles by at least one-quarter. One American procedure, the use of the automobile safety belt, has found some welcome in Japan. Dr. McFarland, of Harvard University, devised this belt on the basis of hints he took from similar belts used in aircraft.

In spite of these things, however, accidents on the road continue. The causes are various. In 1972, during the long holiday that takes places in Japan from the end of April to the first week in May, the national police conducted a research study on deaths caused by automobiles being driven for leisure purposes and discovered that nearly two-thirds of them occurred on the way home. Speeding was the first cause; it was followed, in this order, by drunken driving, overfatigue, and dozing. In short, the usual things. It turned out that in many cases the attention of the driver had been diverted from duty by friends or sweethearts. Interestingly, in America, etiquette is strict on these matters. For instance, people in the automobile do not talk un-necessarily to the driver. Even if one of the passengers is sleepy, he stifles his yawns, because they are infectuous and might cause the driver to become sleepy too.

Taxi Company, Case Number One: My first work with a taxi company began in January, 1967, when Mr. Shigeo Horie, of the Taito Office of the Kokusai Auto-mobile Company, got in touch with me. After discussions, we decided to institute a two-month preparations period. Then we moved into full implementation of a bio-rhythm system. Immediately traffic accidents involving the taxis of this company dropped by 30 percent. They continued to decrease until, by 1971, they had fallen to 50 percent of their former level. During the preparations period, we did not gave the drivers biorhythm calendars. This was done on the basis of the behavioral-science theory that nothing has less effect than something regarded superstitiously as magical protection. At the same time, we used the period to help the drivers under-stand the meaning of biorhythm and to show them that they were to employ biorhythm as a scientific method of self-control.

   Each year, from 50 to 60 percent of all taxi accidents occur on drivers' sensitivity caution days. Reasons for this include the long periods during which the drivers are confined in their vehicles, traffic congestion, and stresses arising from troubles caused by passengers. Obviously, a sound approach to mental hygiene alone would be sufficient to reduce the number of accidents brought on by these factors.

   Mr. Jinpei Suzuki, who was in charge of safety work, said that, for a period, drivers newly entering the company were not scheduled to work on their caution days. As a consequence of this policy, new drivers were able to maintain no-accident records. This is a good idea. Although biorhythm is a tool in autogenic training, labor hygiene must be applied in the first few months of adaptation to a new work environment, since fatigue is likely to be great during this time.

Taxi Company, Case Number Two: The following were the main points in the biorhythm guidance program instituted for the Miyago Tourist Taxi Company in Aomori, Aomori Prefecture. (1) Free distribution of materials and devices for the program to all drivers and thorough instruction on the nature of biorhythm and the ways in which to use the devices. (2) Institution of a merit program. The goal was established for the entire company of one million kilometers of travel without accident or traffic violation of any kind. After this goal was attained, certificates of achievement were awarded for each additional ten thousand kilometers of accident-free travel. An accident caused by any one of the company's drivers would reduce the accident-free milage of the entire company to zero, and the cycle would have to begin again. The system was a great success. Not long after its implementation in October, 1971, the company reached its initial goal and has since established new goals.

   Masao Osanai, resident instructor of the Japan Biorhythm Laboratory in Aomori, has carried the program to electrical companies, factories, offices, financing firms, and department stores with remarkable success.

Telephone and Telegraph Company: The Yokohama Municipal Controls Division discovered that of 28 accidents in city offices for the year 1966, 2.2 times as many occurred on caution days of personnel as on noncaution days. Of thirty-six instances of mistakes in telegrams, twenty-two occurred on caution days of workers. These high rates led to the implementation of a biorhythm system to reduce mistaken deliveries and traffic accidents in the Yokohama North Telephone and Telegraph Office. For one year after the implementation, no accidents occurred, and at present the rate has dropped by from one-quarter to one-third the former level. This success has led to the introduction of the system in telegraph and telephone offices throughout the nation.

At the time of the introduction of the system at the Yokohama North bureau, red and yellow tacks were put over the name plates of delivery personnel when they had caution and semicaution days. Later, to prevent lapsing into mechanical habit, Thursdays were established as traffic safety days. On these days, small triangular flags bearing Japanese words meaning Safety-publicity Vehicle were attached to the front wheels of the delivery personnel's bicycles. These flags serve as successful devices in individual autogenic training. On noncaution days, the flags are green. On caution days they are red, and on semicaution days they are yellow. Not a single deliveryman has requested to be relieved from duty on his caution days.

The good results of this program have influenced the safety programs of all of Kanagawa Prefecture, in which Yokohama is located. For instance, stimulated by this program, the Traffic Safety Center of the prefectural police headquarters conducted a study of the suitability of its drivers on the basis of information for the years between 1968 and 1970. They coordinated data on 189 people involved in 411 accidents with information on the biorhythms of these same people, and learned that of all the accidents, 260 (64.4 percent) occurred on caution days.

The suitability investigation dealt with three factors: intellect, emotional stability, and motor agility. It was learned that intellect is totally unrelated to accidents on caution days. The greater the emotional instability of the person, the larger the number of accidents in which he is involved. People who are normal in terms of motor agility tend to cause fewer accidents. The value of the finding concerning emotional stability is doubled when biorhythm is employed as a means of autogenic training in programs for traffic safety.

Age probably has much to do with the low rate of accidents among people who are normal in terms of motor agility. Since younger people tend to drive faster, it is difficult to determine definite relations between motor agility alone and traffic accidents.

Investigations conducted by the State of Connecticut, in the United States, reveal interesting facts about traffic accidents and age. The state investigation panel found that, as age increases, the number of traffic-caused deaths decreases: 1.5 for every 100,000 miles traveled in the age group from 16 to 21; 1 for the same milage in the age group between 22 and 27; 0.7 in the group between 28 and 47; and 0.6 in the group between 48 and 65. Older people are more cautious and drive more slowly. When they encounter a sudden emergency condition, however, their reduced motor agility makes them less likely than younger people to react fast enough to save themselves. The ability to react to changing light conditions is a case in point.

Specialists agree that this ability begins to decrease after the age of forty and decreases remarkably after the age of fifty. This means that the older person who is deliberately driving carefully may be involved in an accident because of his inability to adapt to such things as bright oncoming headlights or to other demands of twilight and nighttime driving.

Personality too affects the frequency with which individuals are involved in accidents and other unpleasantness. The egoist who is prone to fights, the person who is in court for other reasons as well as for traffic violations, and the person who is antisocial and irresponsible are all likely to cause accidents. Autogenic training and biorhythm study can help these people and can allow them to contribute to the development of a more pleasant environment in their places of work.

Bus Company: Application of biorhythm has enabled the bus department of the Omi Railways Nagahama office to set a record of five million kilometers without accident. This and the improvements made in the working environment of this company by autogenic training are famous both in Japan and in other nations. Five million kilometers is equal to seven round trips between the earth and the moon, or much more distance than was traveled by the Apollo spacecraft, on which scientific knowledge, time, and money were lavished.

Autogenic Training in the Reduction of Accidents: About ten years ago, the German police officer Max Steves published a report in a national police journal on the biorhythm conditions of drivers involved in 1,200 traffic accident. He discovered that, of the total, 649 (54 percent) occurred on the caution days of the drivers. This means that traffic accidents occur from three to four times more frequently on caution as on noncaution days. Steves further analyzed relations between accidents and plus and minus biorhythm phases and showed that they are less influential than the relations with caution days. When all three cycles are negative, accidents occur with twice as great a frequency as when all three are positive. Nonetheless, the figures for minus and plus phases were much lower than those for caution days. Accidents occurred with only three times as great frequency when two of the three cycles were negative as when two of them were positive. This shows that attention to the caution days alone is sufficient, if combined with autogenic training, to intensify safety awareness.

Max Steves did not develop high-level discussions of this kind. He only analyzed accidents and showed that, because of their influence on such occurrences, biorhythm can be useful in safety programs. He did not suggest ways in which they could be useful.

It is not surprising that, when the news of the dramatic reduction in traffic accidents resulting from the application of my biorhythm and autogenic-training system was made public throughout the world, the very first requests I received for material on the subject came from the German magazine *Bunte* in December, 1970.

At this point, I should like to discuss a few accidents that have occurred in Japan and that caused great stir in the news media. I shall pay special attention to accidents involving death.

Death of the World Flyweight Champion Boxer Masao Oba (born on October 21, 1949): At eleven thirty on the morning of January 25, 1973, Oba, while driving a 1973 Chevrolet Corvette on Line Five of the Tokyo Municipal Express Highway, crossed a center-line barrier twenty-five centimeters high at a large curve, in an area called Edobashi, and crashed into an oncoming, eleven-ton truck in the opposite lane. The automobile was crushed, and Oba was killed instantly. Police investigations showed that he had been traveling at nearly one hundred kilometers an hour. Unable to make the left curve, he zigzagged, lost control of the car, crossed the center barrier, and collided with the truck.

A boxer with highly developed motor nerves, he should have been able to react fast to an emergency of this kind. The automobile was both new and of high performance capabilities. The only possible conclusion is that Oba himself made a fatal mistake. His biorhythm chart for that day reveals the shocking condition in which all three cycles are in caution days.

On March 4, 1971, a young truck driver with the same triple accumulation of caution days was involved in a serious incident at the Fuji Express Railways intersection in the city of Fuji Yoshida. The small truck he was driving collided with a train on the tracks. The train, which was traveling at a speed of sixty kilometers an hour, derailed and overturned. Fifteen people were killed, and seventy-two were injured. After the accident, the driver told the following story.

"When I reached the intersection, the barrier was already down; and the warning bell was ringing. Wind had shaken loose some of the load of plywood in the back of my truck. I got out of the cab and walked around to the rear to adjust it. But I forgot to put on the handbrake. The truck began moving suddenly, broke through the barrier, and collided with the train."

(upper) Automobile accident involving Masao Oba. (lower) Driver of the truck that collided with a train on the Fuji Express Railway

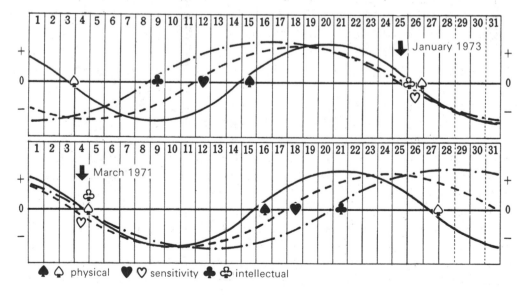

♠ ♤ physical   ♥ ♡ sensitivity   ♣ ♧ intellectual

These two classic cases clearly show the relation between biorhythm conditions and accidents. But, as should have been made clear in the discussion of materials published in the German newspaper journal, information of this kind is not enough to make biorhythm study a constructive, meaningful factor in accident prevention. To do this, a practical system must be developed. To answer the need, I have worked out a system combining biorhythm with autogenic training. I shall now cite one example of its use from a report by Masao Osanai, the resident representative of the Japan Biorhythm Laboratory in Aomori Prefecture. The report was published in the *Biorhythm News*, which is distributed to all members at the annual summer conference of the Japan Biorhythm Laboratory, and in the *Biorhythm Report, 1973*.

"Yokichi Daidoguchi, president of the Miyago Tourist Taxi Company (40 vehicles and 85 employees) met with me for a discussion of traffic safety. For some time, I have been investigating the possibility of using biorhythm in accident reduction. As the outcome of our talks, he decided to implement a biorhythm accident-prevention program in his company in 1971. He set a goal of one million kilometers of travel by his company personnel without accident and without traffic violation of any knid.

"In concrete terms, the program consisted of the following.

1. Distribution of biorhythm calendars to all employees and the institution of a course to explain biorhythm to them.

2. Guidance in the preparation of biorhythm calendars.

3. Institution of a program of a goal of one million kilometers of accident-free traffic-violation-free driving and awarding of certificates of achievement for each ten thousand miles of safe driving.

4. Establishment of the ruling that a violation or accident on the part of any member of the staff would return the entire company record to zero and necessitate a fresh start for the entire group.

5. Miscellaneous points.

"The plan was instituted in the middle of October, 1971. In the first phase, when we merely distributed the calendars and held lectures to explain biorhythm, the number of accidents did not diminish, though the drivers of the company were usually the victims, not the perpetrators, of the accidents that occurred. By the middle of October, we had finished a course of instruction in the preparation and use of biorhythm calendars for the entire staff. The final day of the course of lectures was the first day in the campaign for one million kilometers of safe driving. A bulletin board was put on the wall of the drivers' lounge. On the board were posted the number of kilometers of driving for the given day and the accident status to date. In a period of ten days, the drivers had already driven ten thousand kilometers without unpleasant incident. The officer in charge of accidents in the company had the following remarks to make.

" Accidents stopped almost as if by magic. Before this, every other day I got reports of crashes or collisions over the radio. Then those reports stopped. I had been buried under work connected with dealing with accidents and their aftermath. Suddenly that kind of work vanished. I even began to feel a little odd about having nothing to do. But all the drivers became happier. Our place of work turned into a place of laughter. It was easier for me to give instructions about work. I never dreamed that biorhythm could have such an effect. "

Osanai made the following conclusions about his experience.

"Biorhythm acts like a medicine for the mind. Ways of using and compounding this medicine must be devised for each individual case. Application of them in commercial organizations demands the following conditions.

"The head of the organization must master a certain amount of knowledge about biorhythm: he must understand this theory and application and must know the ways to prepare biorhythm calendars.

"All of the officers in the company must have the same degree of knowledge, which can be acquired in two or three hours of lectures.

"All of the company employees must be informed to the same degree and must be instructed on ways to use their knowledge in self-control programs.

"These three conditions must be fulfilled. I have reached this conclusion as a consequence of three years of work with transportational facilities, factories, offices, financing organizations, and department stores. In addition to experimental work with organizations of this kind, I have enjoyed advice from Professor Tatai and have attempted to put that advice to practical use.

"To take care of everything related to a traffic accident amounting to actual damage costs of ten thousand yen requires an outlay of fifty thousand yen (according to an investigation by the Aomori Branch of the Tohoku Electric Power Company). To make a pure profit of fifty thousand yen under conditions imposed by such an accident demands that the organization make a gross sale of five hundred thousand yen, if pure profit is taken to mean ten percent of total business showings. This single example shows how immense the costs of an accident can be and how negative its effects are on business. These effects are magnified when the accident involves loss of life as well as loss of property.

"When business, for instance, as shown on a graph, seems to be progressing well, losses resulting from mismanagement are still more important. I am convinced that biorhythm acts like a medicine to cure such personnel management problems, though in the past they have been considered incurable."

In concluding this chapter, speaking from the standpoint of a health designer, I should like to make the following suggestions to drivers.

1. Take good care of your stomach and intestines, because trouble in these organs disturbs the integrity of the autonomous nervous system and might cause dizziness and nausea, which in turn greatly lower driving abilities. Have fixed hours for meals and engage in sports or take walks to keep your stomach and intestines in good condition.

2. On caution days in the physical cycle, pay special attention to speed limits because, at such times, the motor nerves are dull and accidents are likely to occur. Even if you are not drinking, consider your condition to be that of a person who has taken a moderate amount of alcohol.

3. On caution days in the emotional cycle, do not pass other automobiles. At these times, when you are likely to be irritable, competition, upsets in relations with other people, and quarrels are to be avoided at all costs.

4. On intellectual-cycle caution days, pay special attention to pedestrian cross-

ings and other signals and signs. At such times, the attention tends to wander. In many instances, this results in short braking, which causes whiplash injuries.

5.   Do not take cold medicines or tranquilizers because they lower driving performance and tend to cause accidents.

6.   If you feel tired or sleepy, even in the middle of a trip, rest. In the United States, the rule is that no person drive for more than one and one-half hours at a stretch. Especially in the case of holiday driving, make certain that you get enough rest beforehand and that you eat nourishing foods.

7.   Do not drive on an empty stomach because lowering of blood sugar often leads to driving mistakes. Keep honey, candy, or chocolates on hand in the automobile at all times. The Americans use chewing gum for this purpose.

8.   People with high blood pressure or heart trouble should not drive. They may cause accidents. But, in addition, the stress of driving in heavy traffic can shorten their lives.

9.   People suffering from rheumatism or asthma should not drive on days when the weather is uncertain. Though they are not aware of bodily upsets, they may be subject to latent insecurities that, like caution days, can cause driving mistakes.

10.   Drivers must not be drinkers. Driving even after the effects of alcohol have apparently worn off is dangerous. In England, investigation has shown that people who tend to have a low level of blood sugar often cause accidents when under the influence of alcohol. After a moderate amount of drinking, do not drive for at least ten hours.

Train Accidents, Crimes, and Suicides

The caution days of many people must be investigated in cases of large-scale train accidents. In other words, when teamwork is not as good as it ought to be, large accidents can occur. Some people claim that physical rhythms are of the utmost importance in cases of crime and suicide. It seems that counseling for people with tendencies to such things must be timed to the positive phases of the emotional cycle.

The engineer **Früh,** who was a follower of Dr. Fliess, developed a number of tools for use with biorhthym study and wrote several books on the subject. As I have already said, his work is too mechanical and too much play with numbers to convince me completely. Nonetheless, some of the examples he cites are excellent reference material.

Train Accidents: On February 18, 1947, occurred a major collision on the Pennsylvania Railway. In the accident, 22 people were killed and 139 injured. The losses

Collision between a truck and a train on the Fuji Express Railway

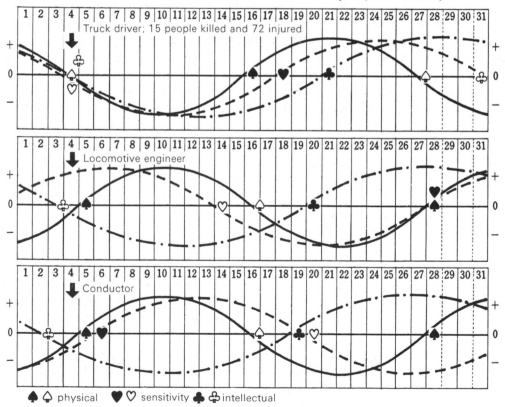

♠ ♤ physical ♥ ♡ sensitivity ♣ ♧ intellectual

amounted to a staggering two million dollars in the money of the time. It turned out that the engineer and his three assistants were all experiencing caution days.

On April 19, 1949, the keeper of an intersection gate on a Swiss railway neglected to lower the barrier. A bus collided with a train, resulting in numerous deaths and injuries. This and two similar accidents at interesection gates (Friedrichshafen, July 7, 1959; Winterthur, February 11, 1970) took place on days when the gate keepers were experiencing caution days in their physical and sensitivity cycles and negative phases in their intellectual cycles.

There are other cases—like the accident that took place on a Berlin express line, killing twenty-two people—in which conductors, though unaware of it, were controlled by their caution day conditions. The engineer of the Swiss train that, on July 21, 1971, failed to make a curve while traveling at a speed of 140 kilometers an hour, was experiencing semicaution days in his physical and sensitivity cycles and a negative phase in his intellectual cycle.

The driver of the light truck that collided with an express train at the town of Fuji Yoshida in 1971 (see details on p. 91) was experiencing one of those disastrous times that occur only once or twice a year when all three cycles are in caution days. The charts on p. 91 show the poor biorhythm conditions of the motorman of the electric cars and the conductor on that day. In the light of these calendars, it is scarcely surprising that the conductor complained that the cord of the hand emergency brake snapped when he pulled it.

On October 25, 1971, a serious head-on collision took place in a tunnel on the Kintetsu Railways in Japan; 25 people were killed, and 237 were injured. Of course, the fact that the train operates on a single line in this particular zone is the fundamental cause of the tragedy. But the initial cause was abnormal operation of the ATS (automatic train stop) system. The motorman of one of the electric cars stopped at the entrance of the tunnel, closed the cock of the airbrake of the locomotive, and began making a spot check. At this time, an assistant from the station, without saying anything about it, released the brake that the motorman had set. Five days after the incident, it was learned that this had been the true cause. The biorhythm conditions of the people involved in this accident show what Dr. McFarland means by an evil conjunction: the motorman was in the negative phase of his sensitivity and intellectual cycles and was experiencing a physical caution day. The assistant who released the brake (he was killed in the accident) was experiencing a sensitivity caution day between physical and intellectual caution days.

During the rush hour on the morning of March 28, 1972, a commuter train standing in one of the large Tokyo stations was bumped from the rear by another train on the same line. A total of 552 people were injured. The driver of the rear train had been distracted by the ATS signal, which rang without stopping. On that day, the driver of the rear train was in a high positive phase in his physical cycle and a negative phase in his sensitivity cycle. He was experiencing an intellectual caution day. The high positive physical phase is probably connected with the accident. He said, "I heard the ATS the minute I pulled into Funabashi Station. I thought it must be a power failure and stopped once. Then, thinking to check the station signal, I decided to pull up. That was when I saw the train parked sixty or seventy meters

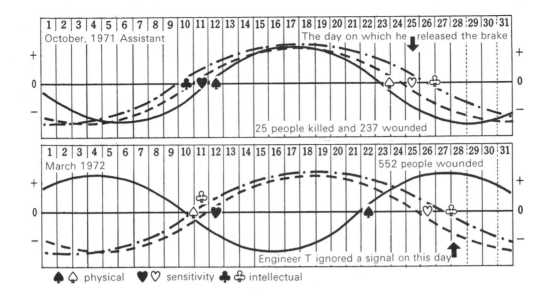

♠ ♤ physical   ♥ ♡ sensitivity   ♣ ♧ intellectual

ahead of me. I pulled the emergency brake, but there was not enough time."

A mistake was made in a basic operation. No matter how exact the mechanical automatic control device, it cannot control human carelessness. This once again points up the significance of the use of biorhythm, which can control human carelessness.

Crimes: Investigations conducted on 50 people involved in armed robberies, murders, battery cases, rape, and other violent crimes showed that 2.5 times as many such acts occur on sensitivity caution and semicaution days as on noncaution days and that 4.7 times as many occur when the intellectual cycle is in the negative phase as occur when it is in the positive phase. Since the complications of biorhythm demand examinations of at least three hundred cases, this set of data cannot be regarded as in any way final.

A notorious crime series occurred in 1968 in Japan. A man killed a guard at a famous Tokyo hotel. Later he shot a policeman at the Yasaka Shrine in Kyoto. He then shot a taxi driver in Hakodate and another taxi driver in Nagoya, before being arrested at a business school in Tokyo. Using his connections with the police, a doctor of my acquaintance investigated the matter from the biorhythm standpoint and related his findings to me. They reminded me of something once told me by a German doctor: when the physical cycle is in its most positive phase and the sensitivity cycle and intellectual cycle are negative, a person can be capable of great violence. As the calendar on p. 94 shows, the criminal in the multimurder case was experiencing an intellectual caution day, a positive physical, and a negative sensitivity cycle at the time of his first crime. He was experiencing negative sensitivity and intellectual cycles and a physical caution day at the time of his second crime and a physical caution day and a semicaution intellectual day and a positive sensitivity cycle at the time of the third crime. At the time of the fourth crime, one day after his sensitivity caution day, he was in a highly positive physical- and intellectualcycle condition. On the day of his arrest he was experiencing a sensitivity caution day,

Biorhythm condition of the criminal discussed on pp. 93–94

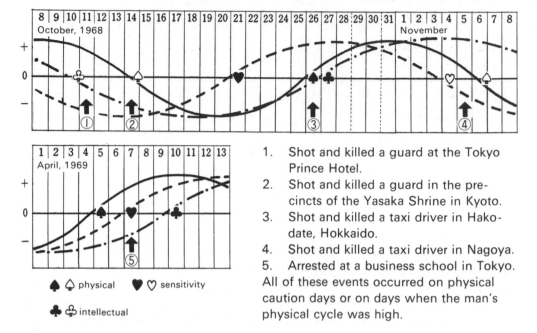

1. Shot and killed a guard at the Tokyo Prince Hotel.
2. Shot and killed a guard in the precincts of the Yasaka Shrine in Kyoto.
3. Shot and killed a taxi driver in Hakodate, Hokkaido.
4. Shot and killed a taxi driver in Nagoya.
5. Arrested at a business school in Tokyo.

All of these events occurred on physical caution days or on days when the man's physical cycle was high.

♠ ♤ physical   ♥ ♡ sensitivity   ♣ ♧ intellectual

a positive physical and a negative intellectual day. Of the five days on which incidents occurred, four were caution days.

Suicides: A number of cases of suicides among famous writers point up the importance of biorhythm conditions in relation to this drastic act, regarded as criminal in some parts of the world, though not in Japan. For instance, the Japanese novelist Osamu Dazai killed himself on June 13, 1948, at a time when he was experiencing an intellectual caution day, a positive physical phase, and a negative sensitivity phase. Ernest Hemingway shot himself with a rifle on July 2, 1961, when he was experiencing a sensitivity caution day and positive phases in both physical and intellectual cycles. On September 21, 1972, the novelist and dramatist Henri de Monteran shot himself with a pistol; he was seventy-six at the time. According to his secretary, he had been gravely worried about losing his sight. When he died, he was experiencing a mid-cycle physical caution day and negative phases in both his sensitivity and intellectual cycles.

The famous motion-picture director Akira Kurosawa, whose prize-winning *Rashomon* brought the Japanese film industry into worldwide prominence after World War II, attempted to kill himself on December 22, 1971. At the time, he was experiencing a negative phase in his physical cycle and a mid-cycle sensitivity caution day. The following day was his intellectual mid-cycle caution day. He was sixty-one. Possibly biorhythm conditions play an important part in leading artistic people to kill themselves when they reach an age when they begin to fear the loss of their creative powers.

Ashihei Hino, author of a novel called *Wheat and Soldiers*, killed himself on

Biorhythm conditions of famous people on the days on which they planned or committed suicide

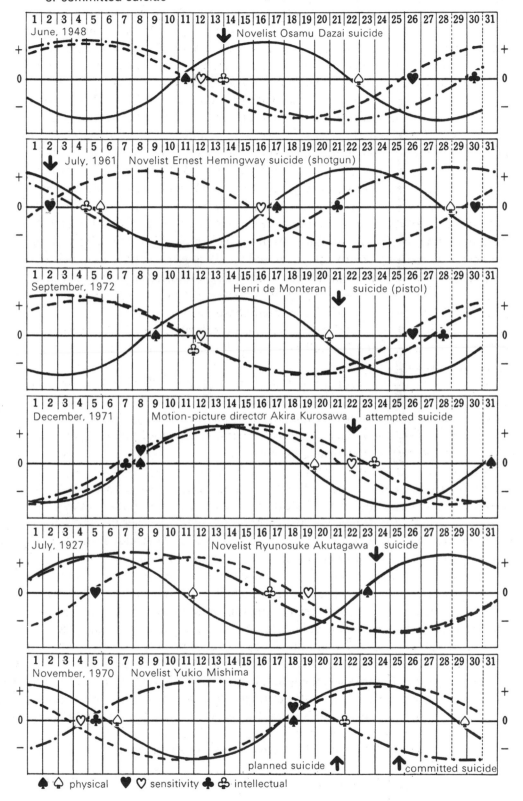

♠ ♤ physical   ♥ ♡ sensitivity   ♣ ♧ intellectual

January 23, 1960, when he was experiencing semicaution days in both his physical and intellectual cycles and a positive phase in his sensitivity cycle. Ryunosuke Akutagawa, another famous author, killed himself early on the morning of July 24, 1927; he was experiencing a caution day in his physical cycle and minus phases in both his sensitivity and intellectual cycles. On June 9, 1923, Takeo Arishima and a woman journalist committed suicide together. He was experiencing a caution day in his sensitivity cycle and a semicaution day in his intellectual cycle.

Nobel Prize winner Yasunari Kawabata, who was born on June 11, 1899, was discovered dead from suicide on the night of April 17, 1972. At the time, his sensitivity and intellectual cycles were positive; and his physical cycle was negative, a combination that is precisely suited to the nature of a mature literary artist.

On November 25, 1970, in a room in the eastern headquarters of the National Self-defense Forces, in Tokyo, the novelist Yukio Mishima committed ritualistic suicide by *harakiri*. His death is thought by some to have influenced the suicide of Yasunari Kawabata. Information has been made public to establish the fact that Mishima made the decision to kill himself on November 21 of the same year. He was then experiencing positive physical and sensitivity phases and an intellectual caution day. On the day of the actual suicide, he manifested the condition that has already been referred to as likely to lead to violent action: positive physical and sensitivity phases and negative intellectual phase.

Once again, in the light of these data, it is necessary for me to emphasize the fallacy of believing that all is well as long as physical, sensitivity, and intellectual cycles are positive.

Many causes are given for suicides: weariness of the world and of living, sickness, psychological abnormality, family troubles, poverty, and unhappy love affairs. Weariness of living accounts for the largest number of successful cases of suicide (one-quarter of the total). But unhappy love affairs account for the largest number (again, one-quarter) of the unsuccessful cases.

From the standpoint of the study of suicide, however, none of these apparent causes is a cause at all; they are all only circumstances. When a normal person feels moved to kill himself, two mental attitudes must be at work simultaneously: the present is a time of suffering, and the future is hopeless. Neither the first nor the second cause is sufficient alone to lead a person to commit suicide instantly. Statistics make it clear that the numbers of suicides decrease in time of war.

It must be remembered that the repressive force instinctive to the human being is always at work. It is the predicament in which Hamlet finds himself when he says, "To be or not to be." For this very reason, on caution days, when this ambivalent character is even stronger, it is only natural that accidents, crimes, and suicides should increase. At such insecure times, the moral of respect for life, which manifests maximum repressive force, is of great significance. As I have repeatedly emphasized from the opening of this book, the ultimate goal of biorhythm study is to enable you to employ this respect for life—without reference to theories—as a technique for living. People who are aware of the need for respect for life should be able to reduce accidents on caution days and ordinary days as well.

The test on pp. 98–99 for lethal behavior will serve as reference in judging the degree to which you are capable of violence. Capability of violence means the same thing as lethal behavior. It reveals whether it is easy for the person involved to cause accidents or commit violence or suicide.

First, make circles by the numbers adjacent to the entries in group 1 that apply to you. Add the numbers you have circled. Next, make circles by the applicable entries in groups 2 and 3. Add the scores of each group and combine them, taking care to notice that the entries in group 3 are negative numbers. Next multiply the total for group 1 by the result of combining the scores for groups 2 and 3. Notice that the judgment scales at the bottom of the page are marked S for positive and A for negative. If the product of combining groups 2 and 3 is a positive number, use scale S; if it is a negative number, use scale A. S numbers are for introverts and A numbers for extroverts.

Low scores are desirable on this test. If you use your biorhythm techniques skillfully, in a year, you can lower your score on this test by more than ten points. If you notice no reduction in your score in a year, you are not using your biorhythm techniques properly.

Application for Counseling: The West German specialist K. Kämmerle investigated the biorhythm conditions of 1,000 cases of suicide and learned that in from 70 to 80 percent the intellectual phase was negative and the physical cycle was in a caution day or all three cycles were negative. If they can be applied to other peoples as well as to the Germans, his findings could contribute to the generation of a worldwide movement for the prevention of suicide.

The English physiotherapist and hypnotherapist Thomas Barlow produces excellent results by investigating his patients' biorhythm conditions and using his findings in treatment. He has learned that patients who are allowed to chose the time at which they will stop smoking or go on a reducing diet, choose positive biorhythm sensitivity phases in 80 percent of all cases. He has had great success timing treatment according to this kind of consideration. Reports of such success suggest that biorhythm sensitivity conditions are important in counseling. Generally, it is correct to assume that people are more cooperative when their sensitivity cycle is in the positive phase.

Make circles around the number of the entries that apply to you and total the scores.

Group 1	score
Do not get along well with friends	+2
Careless and hasty	+1
Change your mind often	+1
Conscious of your duty to others	+1
Lack faith	+3
Sleep irregular hours	+1
Eat at irregular times	+1
Get almost no exercise	+1
Uninterested in war news	+2
Concerned about growing old	+2
Changed job or position in the past year	+1
Experienced domestic upsets in the past year	+1
Work does not go as you want it to	+2
Trouble in your love affairs	+2
Home life does not go as you want it to	+3
Daily life is difficult	+3
Suffering from illness	+3
Insecure about progress in work	+2
Business has failed	+3
Suffered a breakup in a love affair	+3
Losing physical strength	+2
Sick and weakly	+3
No hope of an increase in income	+2

Total of group 1 ☐

Group 2

Able to tolerate unpleasantness	+1
Take losing very hard	+2
Easily deceived by others	+2
Moderate in all things	+1
Fond of quiet colors and unflashy things	+1
Fret over failures	+2
Pay little attention to newspaper articles about violent crimes	+1
Not strongly sexually motivated	+1

Group 3

Immediately complain when someone does something you do not like	−2
Become angry easily	−1
Skillful at convincing others	−1
Restless unless leading others	−2
Fond of flashy things	−1
Do not worry about mistakes	−2
Read articles about violent crimes with interest	−1
Strongly motivated sexually	−1

Total of groups 2 and 3 ☐

Judgment:
LTB susceptible, if combination of groups 2 and 3 is *positive*, and its grede is very high (100 and over scores), high (99–80), moderate (79–50), mild (49 and less).
LTB resistant, if combination of groups 2 and 3 is *negative*, and its grade is very high (100 and over scores), high (99–80), moderate (79–50), mild **(49 and less)**.
Remark: The score means (group 1 total) × (combination of **groups** 2 and 3).

Death and Birth

In this chapter, I shall use material from several sources and examples given by a number of famous doctors in order to explain relations between biorhythm and fatal illness and the influence of biorhythm on childbirth. For a long time, dentists, surgeons, and medical practitioners have employed knowledge of biorhythm to prevent sudden drastic worsening of patients' conditions. There are some people today who claim that biorhythm can be used to predict whether a child will be male or female.

As I have already said, Dr. Fliess was motivated by the knowledge that sicknesses tend to develop and people tend to die on caution days. In his time, medical science was not as far advanced as it is now. Many women died of puerperal fever, which occurs at childbirth. Though this is a highly infectuous disease, about 30 or 40 percent of fatal cases occurred on caution days.

Furthermore, a number of other conditions that doctors find it impossible to predict tend to occur on caution days: operations that do not go as expected, excess hemorrhage, unusual effects from anesthetics, unexpected postoperative hemorrhage, death because of clogged blood vessels, recurrent symptoms, and so on. Latent psychological instability tends to cause accidents to occur on caution days. Consequently, today in Europe, many doctors, especially surgeons, include examinations of biorhythm conditions in diagnoses. Among them are Dr. Fritz Wehrli of the Villa Montana Clinic, who included biorhythm in his practice after being introduced to it by Dr. Bodmer, a friend of the famous surgeon Ferdinand Sauerbruch, at Berlin University. He has sent a letter of thanks to engineer Früh reporting that, in two thousand blood transfusions, owing to his use of biorhythm, he has not had a single instant of a patient's suffering serious consequences. Dr. Werner Zabel, of the clinic for biological therapy in Berchtesgaden, examined cases of deaths, postoperative hemorrhage, and obstructions of local anesthetics and found that such things occur more readily on caution days. He says that avoiding surgery on the caution days of patients has greatly reduced accidents and other unpleasant occurrences. It is only natural that European dentists who wanted to take good care of their patients employed biorhythm before World War II. At the ninth conference of the Japan Biorhythm Laboratory, held in Tokyo, in the summer of 1976, dental surgeon Hiroshi Tani reported that, in 700 patients, bad aftereffects occurred in 80 percent of all cases in which teeth were extracted on caution days. No unpleasant aftereffects occurred in 99 percent of patients on whom similar surgery was performed on noncaution days. Of the patients who came to his clinic for treatment of abscess, 80 percent were experiencing caution days at the time. Furthermore, of these, the majority were experiencing physical-cycle caution days.

At the seventh International Interdisciplinary Cycle Research Symposium, held in

West Germany, in 1976, Adolf Kärcher reported on four years of observing his own physical conditions. During that period, out of 1,461 days, he had been in poor physical condition for 59 days, of which 43 had been caution days in the physical or sensitivity cycles. This means that 72.9 percent of his unwell days were caution days. This was much higher than the 27 percent expected in such cases. He also reported on investigations of 400 elderly people between the ages of 60 and 94. In their cases, caution days are of less significance than negative phases in the physical and sensitivity cycles. At such periods, from two to three times as many illnesses, worsenings of symptoms, and deaths occur as in the positive phases of the same cycles. Elderly people ought to take special care on physical caution days, since, as their physical strength fails, the difference between the positive and negative phases of this cycle tend to minimize.

No Need to Worry about Operations: One of the works by Früh, the famous Swiss specialist in biorhythm and one of the seniors in the movement to spread its study, bears a title very much like the heading of this section: *Keine Angst vor der Operation.* Dr. Fliess, the pioneer of the PSI theory, and Dr. Hans Schlieper, one of his successors, have all studied the relations between biorhythm conditions and the success or failure of surgery. In one of his books, Dr. Schlieper examined twelve cases of death from injections, loss of blood, transfusions, and thrombosis that he had witnessed in thirty-two years of clinical experience and commented on the importance of biorhythm in all these instances.

Of course, at time of illness, when the mind and the body are weakened, biological conditions are of special significance, notably in connection with the negative and positive aspects of the physical and sensitivity cycles. There is record of a young, healthy man of twenty-six who was operated on for mild tonsillitis on his sensitivity caution day. Hemorrhage would not cease, and he died five days later on his physical caution day. In another instance, a healthy young girl of eight received vaccination at a time when her physical and sensitivity cycles were both in negative phases. Six days later, when she was simultaneously experiencing physical and sensitivity caution days, she was suddenly stricken with paralysis.

As a result of his study of the experiences of tens of Swiss doctors,—Früh has reported that application of consideration of the physical and sensitivity biorhythm conditions of patients could prevent more than 30 percent of all deaths resulting from

A young man, twenty-six years of age, died on his physical caution day, five days after an operation

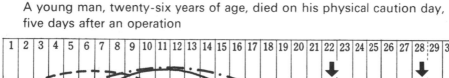

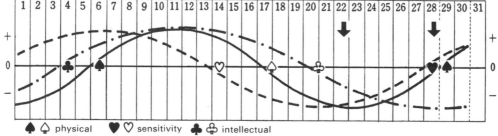

surgical irregularities. In a letter to—Früh, Dr. Wehrli has said that, soon all hospitals will be required to have scales for judging the biorhythm conditions of patients.

Of course, in Japan, where originally biorhythm research was devoted to reducing automobile accidents, we already have the Casio Biolator (see p. 70), which enables us to find out biorhythm conditions instantly without the use of a scale.

As I have already said, I have devoted over thirty years to the study of biological rhythms in the wider sense for the sake of increasing respect for all life in the ecological system of the earth, and especially respect for human life. In the practical field, my efforts have taken the form of work as a health designer.

Even as part of the PSI theory, setting twenty-three days for the physical cycle, twenty-eight days for the sensitivity cycle, and thirty-three days for the intellectual cycle seemed too mechanical at the beginning of my research on the theory.

Fortunately, or unfortunately, since my boyhood, I have been afflicted with occasional attacks of diarrhea brought on by nervousness. After I learned that 78 percent of my attacks of this sickness occur on physical caution days, I saw that biorhythm can be put to use in a daily health-regulation regimen that, in my case, has reduced to half the number of bouts of diarrhea that I suffer. On physical caution days, I take care not to overeat or to drink too much, and I keep regular hours. Although I have not reduced my attacks to zero, I understand what causes them and am able to be calm when they strike because I know that, even without the aid of medicine, they will be cured on the following day.

Here I should like for you to recall the statistical report of Dr. Hans Schwing, of the Swiss National Institute of Technology, who said that the majority of 700 accidents on the job in a series of experiments he made occurred on caution days and that the deaths of 400 cases that he investigated for an insurance company tended to occur on caution days.

Dr. W. von Gonzenbach, director of the Department of Hygiene and Bacteriology of the same Institute of Technology, has said that the most interesting thing in Schwing's doctoral thesis is the way caution days are incorporated. "Caution days are not days when fated, unavoidable accidents or deaths are ordained to occur. By being careful on these days, it is possible to prevent the occurrence of unpleasant incidents. By making it part of a system of mental and physical control, it is possible to find something of practical value in biorhythm."

A few years ago, Henry Le Roy, professor of biological statistics at the Swiss Institute, of Technology, working with Dr. H. Krayenbuhl, chief of the neurosurgery clinic of Zürich University, analyzed 630 cases of accidental death and of heart attack and cerebral apoplexy in terms of the theory of the physical, sensitivity, and intellectual cycles. With important statistical proof, they showed that the physical cycle exercises anespecially strong influence in such cases

Deaths of Famous People: Edward Duke of Windsor died, reportedly of cancer, though this has never been made officially public, in May of 1972. As the graph on p. 103 shows, this was a classic example of a dire event's occurring on the day before one of those days—of which there is usually only less than once a year—when caution days in all three cycles coincide.

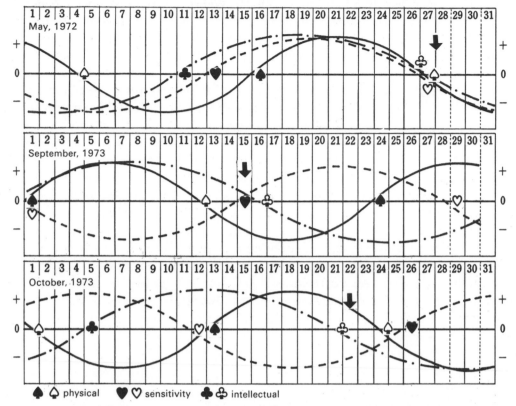

♠ △ physical　♥ ♡ sensitivity　♣ ♧ intellectual

Biorhythm conditions of the Duke of Windsor (top), King Gustav VI (middle) and Pablo Casals (bottom) on the days of their deaths (indicated by arrows)

On September 15, 1973, at the age of ninety-one, King Gustav VI of Sweden, who was both a student of architecture and a specialist in Chinese ceramics, died on his sensitivity caution day. In the same year, on October 22, the world-famous cellist and advocate of freedom and human rights Pablo Casals died on his intellectual caution day. As the cases of these three men suggest, time of death tends to coincide most closely with caution days when the way of life of the person is calm and peaceful. This is because caution days are part of the natural biological system.

The prime minister of Japan during the vital postwar period Shigeru Yoshida

Biorhythm condition of Shigeru Yoshida on the days of his death (indicated by arrow)

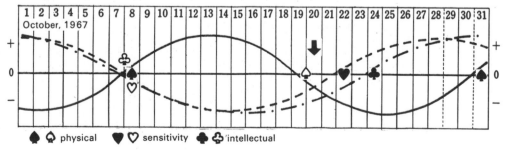

♠ ♤ physical　♥ ♡ sensitivity　♣ ♧ intellectual

caught cold in late September, 1967. An examination of his biorhythm chart in relation to the progress of his sickness shows that he somehow managed to survive the crisis of a triple caution day but succumbed to the next physical caution day, on October 20, when he died of pulmonary paralysis brought on by heart sickness.

Cancer patients who are in the shadow of death sometimes ask me to show them the days on which danger for them is greatest. While feeling sympathy for the patient, I realize that this information can be valuable to them and to their loved ones in making necessary preparations. I generally draw up biorhythm calendars for two months and plot first the physical and then the sensitivity cycles. On several occasions, I have been thanked for the accuracy of my information.

Biorhythm can be of use in predicting births. For instance, if the doctor says that the baby is likely to be born on or about a certain date, it is actually likely to be born on one of the physical or sensitivity caution days shortly before or after that day.

Now to return to the main topic, I should like to call attention to a report made by a group of doctors from the city of Stuttgart who investigated 10,000 patients and found that, in 100 percent of all cases, symptoms were controlled by biorhythm conditions. Adopting a set treatment system for fifteen years, they reduced accidental deaths to zero in a total of over four thousand cases. In so far as possible, they selected times propitious from a biorhythm standpoint in which to perform surgery. This enabled them to prevent deaths from irregularities with anesthetics and blood clots. I have often received telephone calls thanking me for helping chose the correct day on which to perform surgery.

Accidents Involving Famous People: After midnight, on June 28, 1967, while racing along a highway near New Orleans, the famous glamor girl Jayne Mansfield made a driving error. In the next second, her car crashed into a truck in the opposite lane.

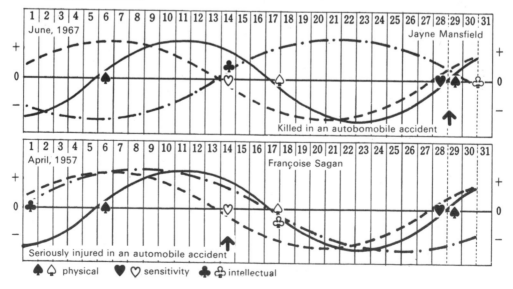

Biorhythm conditions of Jayne Mansfield and Françoise Sagan on the days of their accidents

She was killed instantly. News reports claimed that she had been drinking. Even if she had not, her biorhythm conditions were almost as bad as possible: she was experiencing a physical and a sensitivity caution day and a semicaution day in her intellectual cycle.

The German biorhythm specialist Hugo Max Gross has written that 80 percent of all fatal traffic accidents occur on caution days of the people responsible for them. An accident involving the popular French novelist Françoise Sagan is a case in point. While driving with a friend, on April 14, 1957, she caused an accident in which she received a serious wound. Miraculously, she recovered; but the friend in the car with her was killed. For a novelist, her biorhythm condition was very important because she was experiencing a caution day in her sensitivity cycle. The fact that she was in the positive phase of her physical cycle may have helped account for her miraculous recovery. Hers is an interesting case.

Correlating the information I have received from physicians of long experience, I understand that, on physical caution days, bleeding is severe. This may be an important reason for dentists to avoid such days in extracting teeth.

Biorhythm and Birth: I have already explained what may be called basic medical common sense about the period between the fertilization of the ovum and birth as the source of the individual human life. I have further mentioned the doubt entertained by many medical scientists about the attempt of the engineer Früh to equate the twenty-three human chromosomes and the two hundred and eighty days of the human gestation period with the twenty-three, twenty-eight, and thirty-three days of the human physical, sensitivity, and intellectual biorhythm cycles.

There is no doubt, however, that the instant of birth often occurs on caution days in the mother's physical or sensitivity cycle. For instance, the second child of the English princess Margaret was born on the mother's physical caution day and sensitivity semicaution day. The many other similar cases that could be cited provide valuable food for thought. Früh was an engineer and not a biologist. It is therefore easy to see why he wanted to equate the average two hundred and eighty days of the human gestation period with the twenty-eight-day cycle.

As I have already explained, Naegle's law applies in calculations of dates of birth. This highly accurate method calls for adding seven days to the last menstrual day and subtracting three months. This is based on the scientifically valid fact that fertilization occurs on the ovulation day following the final menstrual day.

In a personal communication, a Canadian doctor has insisted that biorhythm can be used to predict whether a child will be male or female. If fertilization occurs when the physical cycle is positive and the sensitivity cycle negative, the child will be male. It has been empirically, shown that, if the physical cycle is negative and the sensitivity cycle positive, the child will be female. For instance, this was true in the case of the second child of Princess Margaret and has been true in instances of children in the Japanese imperial family.

The Canadian school of thought explains that this theory is correct on the basis of the acid-base proposition of the German gynecologist Franz Unterberger. But not all obstetricians support the explanation. Since I have concentrated on developments in the physical and sensitivity cycles of males and females and have done no research on the ebb and flow of reserve strength of the acidity or alkalinity of blood and other body fluids, I have no definite reason for agreeing with the Canadian school of thought.

Since genetically the numbers of sex chromosomes are the same, at the time of fertilization, the ratio between male and female ought to be the same. But investigations of large numbers of subjects have shown that the actual ratio is 150, or 3 to 2. The number of male infants lost in miscarriages or deaths at birth is overwhelmingly greater than the number of female infants lost as the result of the same causes. Consequently, at birth, the ratio between the sexes is 105; that is, male infants outnumber female infants by only 5 percent. Because more males die young than females by the age of twenty, the ratio between the sexes is equal at the age. But since women live longer than men, in older age groups, females form the larger part of the population.

In this long journey from fertilization to the grave, why the ratio between the sexes should begin at 150 remains an unexplained mystery. The sperm cells determine the sex of the infant. At present, microscopic examination reveals two kinds of sperm cells: the larger ones produce females and the smaller ones males.

The German obstetrician Dr. Rautenstrauch is especially interested in using biorhythm to determine whether a child will be male or female. I met him first in 1975 at a symposium on biorhythm held by him and Adolf Kärcher in West Germany. Our new book *Biorhythm in the World Today, a Data Book*, scheduled for publication in 1978, will present the details of the conclusions mentioned in the report he made at that meeting.

Winning at Sports

Accidents in sports events are likely to be very grave. Drivers in car races are prone to make mistakes if they engage in their sport when their biorhythm conditions are poor. The theory that upsets in the physical cycle are highly influential seems convincing, though in the case of the Japanese, the emotional cycle seems more important. As might be expected, winning and losing in combat sports involving only two participants—wrestling, boxing, and Japanese sumo wrestling—most clearly reflect biorhythm conditions. In the following section, I explain this further on the basis of the experiences of famous boxers and wrestlers.

The reason for the abundance of material on sports and biorhythm is the wide use to which biorhythm methods have been put ever since the coaches and trainers of the German teams in the Berlin Olympics turned their attention to this field in the hope of improving performance. For a long time, coaches and directors of European professional soccer teams have prepared biorhythm charts and have used them in training to strengthen their team members and to enable them to perform at maximum level during meets. Trainers and managers continue to use biorhythm in such endeavors today. An Australian intellectual who once visited Japan informed me that biorhythm had been used in the training of their campion swimmer Miss Shane Gould.

Example One
Obviously all, sportsmen would like to avoid injury; but, since they are involved in tests of skill and strength, accidents do happen and sometimes result in disability or even death. Doctors associated with sports therefore devote much attention to prevention and treatment of injuries caused in accidents. I shall begin my discussion of this field with car racing, which, because of the speed involved, is likely to be the most potentially hazardous of all sports.

The test driver Yukio Fukuzawa was killed instantly at a test course in Shizuoka Prefecture when the Toyota 7 on which he was conducting wind-resistance experiments ran along the course for about 90 meters at a speed of 250 kilometers an hour and crashed into a sign at a curve. The car jumped for another thirty-six meters, and the driver died of a fractured skull and serious burns all over his body. The accident occurred at noon on February 12, 1969. About a week later, the police issued a verdict of probable accidental death caused by a mistake on the part of the driver. The biorhythm calendar of Fukuzawa, who was born in France, on June 18, 1943, showed for the day of his death a double set of semicaution days in the physical and intellectual cycles and a low minus phase in the sensitivity cycle (this calculation

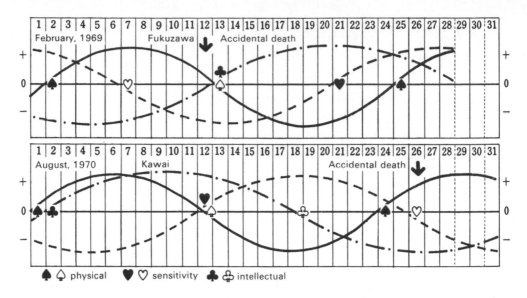

Biorhythm conditions of Yukio Fukuzawa and Minoru Kawai on the days of their deaths

takes into effect the time difference between Japan and France).

At the Suzuka course, on August 27, 1970, the test racer Minoru Kawai, conducting safety tests on a New Toyota 7, crashed into an embankment and died at once of a broken neck and fractured skull. His biorhythm calendar for the day shows that he was experiencing a sensitivity caution day and a high positive physical phase and a low negative intellectual phase (note that this is the imbalance combination in which, according to the chairman of the Swiss Automotive Federation, accidents are most likely to occur).

Similar cases are numerous in Europe as well as in Japan. The noted biorhythm researcher Hugo Gross points out in his book *Biorhythmik* that 80 percent of the many accidental deaths involving racing drivers take place on the caution days of the drivers. It is interesting to note that Adolf Kärcher studied eleven cases of accidental deaths of car racers and learned that, in ten of these cases, the drivers were experiencing a negative physical phase.

In other sports as well, noted athletes, like the boxer Masao Kubo and the famous baseball player Shigeo Nagashima, have been killed or injured during matches or games occurring on their caution days. Obviously health and safety-control programs based on individual biorhythm calendars are of the greatest importance in preventing such serious mishaps. In this connection, a biorhythm calendar with a memorandum column is extremely helpful.

Example Two
Condition is the key to success in sports. It is foolish to try to run at full power all of the time. The best way is to take advantage of strength and talent when the body is in good condition. Trying to maintain the same high pitch all the time is something like gold plating: when stress arises, it will wear away, revealing the base

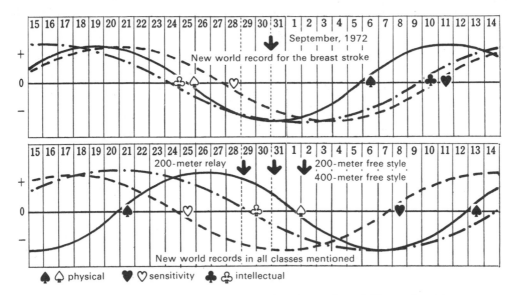

Biorhythm conditions of Nobunori Taguchi (upper) and Shane Gould (lower) on their winning days

metal underneath. To illustrate my meaning, I shall refer to the activities of the Japanese swimming team at the twelfth Olympic Games, held in Munich, in 1972.

Nobunori Taguchi, who set a new world record for the breast stroke and won Japan's first swimming gold metal in the Olympics in sixteen years, adopted a cool attitude. He said that he would win in the second half of the race, and he did. This attitude, supported by low negative phases in all three biorhythm cycles, played an important part in his victory.

Winning jockeys in important Japanese horse races often demonstrate a similar biorhythm condition, proving the fallacy of the simplistic belief that the positive phase is always good and the negative phase always bad.

In addition to power, resoluteness, careful observation of distances with other swimmers, and hard training were advanced as contributive factors in the amazing success of the Australian swimmer Shane Gould, who won three gold medals at the Munich Olympics. When I heard news to the effect that she employs biorhythm in her training, I suspected that this too must have helped her to win and set new world records in spite of occasional apparent slumps.

I have made a chart coordinating some of the most impressive occurrences at the Munich Olympics with the biorhythm conditions of the people involved (p. 110). The column on the far right shows the biorhythm conditions.

Example Three
Research that I have conducted on the careers of such famous *sumo* wrestlers as the now retired Taiho and Kashiwado reveal that they too were strongly influenced by biorhythm conditions and that the influence is strongly apparent in the more experienced wrestlers. But, as I have stressed in the main part of this book, experi-

Light and Dark at the Munich Olympics

athlete	episode	P	S	I
Eddie Hart (U.S.A.)	appeared in the first preliminaries on August 31; disqualified in the second preliminaries	×	×	×
Reynaud Robinson (U.S.A.)	100 m dash in 9.9 seconds	−	+	×
Robert B. Seagren (U.S.A.)	lost pole-vault finals	×	−	+
Wolfgang Nordwig (East Germany)	new 5m50 record, stopping 17-win streak by the USA	−	−	+
Frank Shorter	September 10; won marathon	−	+	+
Mayumi Aoki (Japan)	September 1; new world record in the woman's butterfly	+	+	+
Heidemarie Rosendahl (West Germany)	August 31; won women's running broad jump	−	+	−
Ulrike Meyfarth (West Germany)	September 4, won woman's running high jump	+	+	−

(× indicates a caution day)

ence and skill will always tell when participants in a match are otherwise unequal, though biorhythm conditions may make all the difference in a match between two men of equal power.

For instance, three years before his retirement from the ring, Taiho was absolutely undefeated. In this part of his career, he probably won regardless of his biorhythm conditions. Two years before his retirement, however, biorhythm influenced his victories and failures more dramatically. From this, I infer that he was physically weakening at that time. In 1971, at the time of his retirement, his biorhythm conditions were especially bad; consequently, he must have sensed an ebbing of strength that inspired him to announce his intention of giving up professional *sumo* wrestling.

Example Four
The requirements of boxing, different from those of *sumo* wrestling, make possible fairly easy biorhythm predictions of victory or defeat. For instance, before a non-title match between two Japanese boxers, I was asked to predict the outcome on the basis of the men's biorhythm conditions. I observed that neither would be experiencing a caution day on the day of the match. Both would be in negative intellectual phases; this meant that their abilities to make correct judgments would be on a par. If their strengths were matched, the one whose physical cycle was positive would have a definite advantage. I predicted that, if the match was a long one, he would win, though it might be possible for the other boxer to win if he managed an early knockout. He did not, and the man with the positive physical cycle lasted longer and won.

A famous Japanese boxer lost his title when he fought a match on a day when

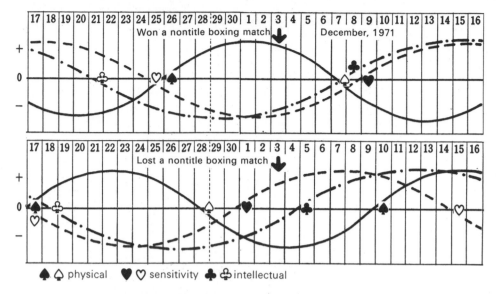

♠ △ physical   ♥ ♡ sensitivity   ♣ ♧ intellectual

Biorhythm conditions of boxers on days of matches

he was experiencing a sensitivity caution day and negative physical and intellectual phases. He had managed to use his special stamina to make an early win on another occasion when he fought on an intellectual caution day and when he was in a positive physical and a negative sensitivity cycle. On still another occasion, when the same boxer was in a disadvantage in terms of biorhythm—intellectual caution day, negative physical cycle, and positive sensitivity cycle—he used autogenic training to help him beat a powerful boxer from another country.

Improving Business Management

Though business methods in Japan differ from those commonly practiced in the West, the following examples of the ways in which application of biorhythm can improve the working environment and assist in sales promotion should be of interest as reference.

The law of moderation is as much a part of the world of nature as biorhythm itself. I am often asked about compatibility for the sake of a better working environment. I always say that people who are too much alike must not be put

Biorhythm conditions of people killed while working on train-track maintenance

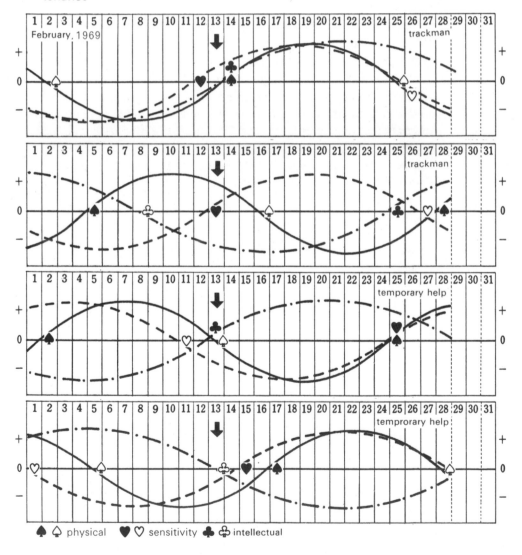

♠ ♤ physical ♥ ♡ sensitivity ♣ ♧ intellectual

together. For instance, if a man and his wife are as similar as twins, they lead an uninteresting life and soon grow tired of each other. If their caution days coincide, the danger of quarrels and accidents doubles.

In 1969, on the Japanese National Railways there occurred a serious accident in which six workers on the tracks were hit by a train and killed. Since no passengers were involved, very little public stir was caused; but the accident was a great shock for the employees and management of the railways and inspired the establishment of a monthly safety day.

The biorhythm conditions of four of the members of the work team are shown in the chart on p. 112. As is obvious from these graphs, if the team had been composed of people whose biorhythm were less similar, the tragedy might have been averted. In the following example, I show a case of a department-store work team whose rates of compatibility were too high for good relations.

In the sensitivity cycle, compatibility should be no higher than 80 percent and no lower than 20 percent.

Department-store Workers: Seven years ago, a certain department store gave me a list of the dates of birth of more than twenty of their employees and asked me to interpret the work team on the basis of biorhythm conditions. I did as I was asked and noticed some characteristic features in connection with compatibility in sensitivity cycles. On the basis of this observation, I made some suggestions that shocked the personnel manager, who acted on my advice at once.

The chart below illustrates my meaning. A and B, both men, are a section head and an assistant section head. C, D, and E are women in their late twenties and early thirties in positions corresponding to those of clerks-in-charge. Each of them has seven or eight younger girls working for her. The sensitivity-cycle compatibility of C, D, and E is as high as can be: 100 percent. Section head **A** maintains a suitable compatibility rate of 70 percent. The compatibility rate between assistant section

A				
7	B			
71	21	C		
71	21	100	D	
71	21	100	100	E

Sensitivity compatibility relations of a group of five people

head B and clerks C, D, and E is 21 percent. That between him and section chief A is a low 7 percent. I could tell from the charts that B was a complete outsider in relation to the rest of the group. The personnel manager of the store told me that such was the case.

This situation corresponds to what Dr. Douglas McGregor, in his book *The Human Side of Enterprise*, refers to as the X theory of management. It is even more important today, when the Y theory of management is being emphasized.

The suitability or lack of it of the personality of the manager is, of course, more important in these situations than biorhythm. But, in departmemt stores, large, unspecified numbers of people work under conditions in which they participate in management only in a low-level way. In such cases, such human cycles as biorhythm exercise a controlling influence on human relations. This in turn strongly affects relations between employees and customers and establishes the reputation of the store for good or bad service. The most important thing for department-store salesgirls to remember is that treatment of customers must project an image of warmth and individuality. For the employee to do this, conditions among all employees sometimes require improving. To this end, biorhythm can be an important aid.

Factory workers often say that they are happiest on the job when they get along well with their fellow-workers. Investigations of human relations among factory workers in the United States bears this out. The research of a specialist has shown that the importance of good relations is especially strong among unskilled and nontechnical laborers. Trouble seems to arise most frequently among groups like young female employees in department-stores. Such trouble may lead to loss of reason for living.

Human beings are not the only creatures that experience difficulty as an outcome of awareness of fellows. Dr. Curt Richter conducted the following experiments on male rats. In a cage he kept first one; then he added another and another, until the group numbered seventeen. After a fixed period, he sacrificed the rats and measured their degrees of stress. As the graph on p. 115 shows, as the number of rats in the cage increased, the weight of the adrenal glands, which are increased by stress, grew steadily, whereas the thymus glands, which are repressed by stress, decreased steadily. I made a study on guinea pigs, animals somewhat more docile than rats, and found the same thing. It is only natural that biorhythm should be useful in increasing on-the-job efficiency and in promoting better employee health. From the standpoint of biorhythm study, it is not surprising that business enterprises and organization in the national Self-defense Forces that have adopted active biorhythm programs should find human relations on the job greatly improved.

Biorhythm affects all human beings. It produces recurring cycles in the body that resemble such meteorological phenomena as fair skies, clouds, rain, and wind. Obviously, in many cases, these phenomena do not manifest themselves openly; but, when they do, the rain and wind metaphorically take the form of accidents, mistakes, and illnesses. Talk about biorhythm conditions among employees on the job creates a strong sense of communion and helps develop an awareness of direct practice of Y-theory management.

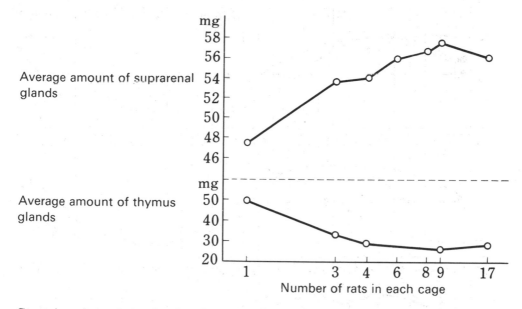

Stress in and population density of rats and their relation to the suprarenal and thymus glands

A foreman at an industrial company in Hiroshima has reported good results from the use of color badges on caution days together with a slogan meaning, "Let's all be aware of each other's biorhythm conditions." The similar badges with different colors for caution days have been effectively employed by the Japanese electric power company.

From a Saleswoman's Notes: On p. 116 is a graphic representation of biorhythm conditions reconstructed from materials in the notes of a qualified beautician and cosmetics saleswoman on three girls who were training under her.

The following points were offered as advice on the basis of what she learned from this investigation. On sensitivity caution days, these steps ought to be observed.

(1) Make memoranda of the things the customer tells you and employ this material in giving advice.

(2) Try to have the customer reevaluate the cosmetics she has used up to the present time.

(3) Talk about the things the customer likes to talk about.

(4) Avoid making pronouncements on your own and let the customer take the lead in the conversation.

(5) Do not act too independently, but treat the customer exactly as you were taught to in training class. This will help you relax.

This particular woman was of a quiet disposition. She found that on days when she was in a positive sensitivity phase, she did well to make deliberate attempts to meet customers she knew to be difficult to convince. When she did her best on such days, she found that she easily met her sales quotas. She learned that this system not only boosted sales, but also promoted good customer relations and, in this way,

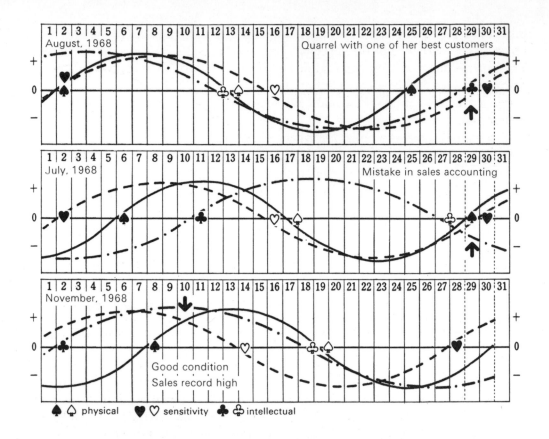

Biorhythm conditions of a cosmetics saleslady

served as excellent advertisement. She devised the following motto, which she repeated to herself daily: "On bad cycle days, smile ten times more than usual. Smile! Smile! Smile!"

The old Chinese saying that there is no danger in a hundred battles for a man who knows his enemy and himself is more than a piece of gnomic wisdom, as the experience of this cosmetics saleswoman, who made positive use of her own biorhythm calendar, proves. As I have repeatedly said, this kind of constant use of the calendar in combination with a memorandum column is of maximum value in autogenic training.

Biorhythm can do more than assist the individual: it can help raise the performance level of entire companies.

A certain Japanese firm greatly increased its efficiency and improved its work atmosphere by taking steps to adapt to biorhythm conditions. For example, older people in the company were warned about drinking or taking hot baths on physical caution days since, at these times, hangovers and cerebral apoplexy can occur more readily than on other days. During positive intellectual and sensitivity phases, salesmen were encouraged to be positive and active; on days in their negative phases, they were warned not to be too eager. On his intellectual caution day, a young man made a serious mistake in a report. He was prepared for a scolding from his superior but was surprised to be let off with an admonition to calm down. On the next day, however, he was called to the superior's office and roundly criticized for his error. The superior finished and then said he had put off the scolding because the day before had been his sensitivity caution day and he realized that, if he chided the employee then, what he said would have been overly emotional and not rationally convincing.

In some instances, personnel managers, observing that a given employee keeps entirely to himself, have investigated the person's biorhythm conditions and have discovered that he is completely incompatible with the others. In such cases, they may solve the problem by transferring the person to a more compatible group.

School Work

Although the rigid and highly demanding system of tests and examinations that Japanese young people must undergo from primary school to university if they want to succeed in scholastic fields is probably unlike anything found in other nations, the way biorhythm can be of assistance to students should serve readers from other countries as reference material concerning the level Japanese biorhythm studies have attained.

The Japanese educator Yoshiyuki Okimura has developed a theory that is of great value to school children. He insists that, in very young children, the nervous and endocrine systems are underdeveloped and that, consequently, the wave movement of the intellectual cycle has not yet manifested itself. He claims that, in dealing with such children, it is recommended to develop educational and safety programs concentrating on the physical and sensitivity cycles and ignoring the intellectual cycle.

On physical and sensitivity caution days, children tend to be sick, sustain injuries, and forget their homework. There is data to indicate that, in addition, they tend to fight, tease small girls or weaker people, and in general work out their resentments and frustrations. In rural areas, at such times, children steal farm produce and make other mischief. In cities, this takes the form of petty thefts and playing with fire.

Of course, they do not do this kind of thing incessantly, for when they become weary they fall asleep, no matter what the time of day. For the sake of their health of mind and body, it is better to concentrate on rest on caution days.

Children of this age group have underdeveloped intellects and are immature in personality. Consequently, until the age of about ten, they should be allowed to live in accordance with natural wave patterns. When they are in their positive phases, they should be encouraged to be active in sports and study. But, when they are in negative phases, they should not be forced. During the negative phases, no attempts should be made to teach them anything new, for such study not only results in no learning, it can also have decidedly detrimental effects. Children require more attention on these matters than adults.

Some of the results of Okimura's study are shown in the following graph of the biorhythm conditions of two children: N, who had a hysterical fit during music class, and H, who had fights with his parents. As is shown, the negative phase exerts a powerful influence. Scolding should be done only during the children's positive phases.

Since the physical cycle controls fatigue, caution is required on the following points.

(1) During the physical negative phase, do not allow children to play until they are very tired.

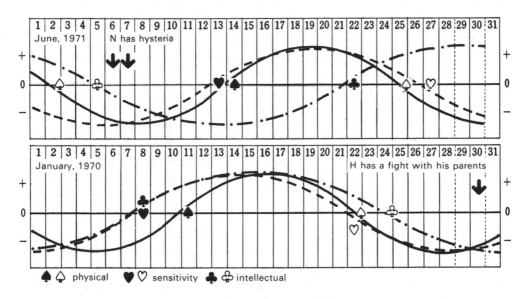

| 1 | 2 | 3 | 4 | 5 | 6 | 7 | 8 | 9 | 10 | 11 | 12 | 13 | 14 | 15 | 16 | 17 | 18 | 19 | 20 | 21 | 22 | 23 | 24 | 25 | 26 | 27 | 28 | 29 | 30 | 31 |

June, 1971   N has hysteria

| 1 | 2 | 3 | 4 | 5 | 6 | 7 | 8 | 9 | 10 | 11 | 12 | 13 | 14 | 15 | 16 | 17 | 18 | 19 | 20 | 21 | 22 | 23 | 24 | 25 | 26 | 27 | 28 | 29 | 30 | 31 |

January, 1970   H has a fight with his parents

♠ ♤ physical   ♥ ♡ sensitivity   ♣ ♧ intellectual

From the data of Yoshiyuki Okimura

(2) Children should finish their studies as early as possible.

(3) The pace of study should be somewhat slower than in the positive phases.

(4) But children should not be allowed to do nothing but play: they must do some study.

(5) Care should be exercised in rationing the amount of time they may spend watching television. They should go to bed early.

(6) When they awaken in the morning feeling fresh, they should be encouraged to study, if even for only ten to twenty minutes.

(7) When children are in negative sensitivity phases, they should not be forced to learn new things but should be allowed to study as they wish.

(8) New materials should be introduced when children are in positive sensitivity phases.

Yoshiyuki Okimura is of the opinion that autogenic training can be initiated with children of more than ten years of age. I believe that results are better if the training is begun on an ordinary caution day and not on a double or triple caution day or a caution day sandwiched between two violently differing positive and negative phases.

For children over ten, emphasis must be placed on the intellectual cycle. Subjects that demand deductive thinking—mathematics, physics, chemistry, and so on—are best studied when the child is in the positive phase. When the child is in a negative intellectual phase, he should study things that involve simple repetitions like languages or things that involve only memorization of facts like history and geography. If these subjects are pursued when the child is in a positive intellectual phase, he will only become bored or tired.

It is not as easy to determine what should and should not be done during the sensitivity positive phase. In general, the high phase is good for attending lectures; but people with extroverted personalities may find it difficult to remain calm, merely sitting and listening. Studying for examinations for such people can be boring.

They should seek relief by such simple changes as studying in a different room.

Introverted people who attempt to study when they are in negative sensitivity phases may become gloomy and insecure. They should try to get over this by doing light exercise or by listening to music. Parents who are observing the study habits of their children must pay attention to these points. For children who are very young, they must ignore the intellectual cycle and concentrate on the sensitivity cycle. On sensitivity caution days, very young children tend to be sleepy, whereas older children, especially those who have reached puberty, are usually unable to sleep.

People of high intelligence are more intensely affected by the differences in negative and positive intellectual phases. Students who consistently make good grades require suitable guidance on the intellectual cycle. People of low intelligence, on the other hand, are as little influenced by positive and negative intellectual phases as very young children, even after they reach their low teens.

It is unnecessary to be too concerned about the differences between the positive and negative phases of the physical cycle in children, though it is important to be on guard to prevent their catching cold or suffering from diarrhea on physical caution days. If a child must take an examination on a physical caution day, care must be exercised on his health control program to see that he does not catch cold or fall asleep while studying. For children with weak stomachs, parents must attempt to provide especially easily digested food for three or four days before caution day. Eggs and cheese are good, and such vegetables as parsley and lettuce are essential because they provide vitamin C, which relieves stress and helps to prevent colds. Of course, vitamins B_1, B_2, B_3, and B_6 must be included in the daily diet because of their helpful influence on the nervous system. Children should be given liver once a week.

When an examination falls on a double—sensitivity and intellectual—caution day, steps must be taken to prevent mishap. If the school is in an unfamiliar place, two or three days before the examination, go there to conduct rehearsals to make certain the child is absolutely familiar with the traffic situation. This will have a calming effect. On the day before, elder brother or father must check the child's materials to ensure that he forgets nothing.

Instruct the child not to rush, but to read each question through completely twice before beginning to answer and to take two deep breaths each time.
Once again, I must remind the reader that it is folly to judge everything on the basis of positive and negative phases. Depending on the personality of the individual, there are cases in which the positive is more disadvantageous than the negative phase. Check the list on p. 61, but be certain that caution days are clearly marked on biorhythm calendars.

Like the work of Freud, the kinds of things that I have been discussing cannot be expressed in terms or mere statistics in a way that would be convincing to all people. On the other hand, statistics alone cannot develop into a science of the individual to the extent that the study of biorhythm can. This is true because human beings are not mass-produced, identical creatures: each is as different in personality as in facial features.

Of course, this does not imply that I am despising basic research in the field. In recent years, Douglas E. Neil and Thomas A. Wyatt, of the American Naval Post-graduate School, conducted basic research on the grades of four young men in fifteen subjects for fourteen months and learned that they did better when their intellectual cycles were in positive phases.

The West German educator Adolf Kärcher studied the grades of students between the ages of 16 and 19 for 6 years and learned that 83 percent of all failures occurred when the intellectual cycle of the individual was negative and that grades tended to drop on intellectual caution days and on days when two of the three cycles were in negative—especially low negative—phases. It is true that these investigations were conducted on only a small number of students. Still they indicate the influence of biorhythm conditions on grades.

From these studies, it is possible to say without a doubt that the intellectual biorhythm cycle influences the grades of students of high-school age or older. Of course, it would not do to ignore the role of the negative phases of the physical and sensitivity cycles in this connection.

Nor is the compatibility ratio between teachers and students to be overlooked. In his book *Denken, Lernen, Vergessen*, Frederic Vester asserts the conviction that learning is more efficient and longer-lasting when the student is on the same wave length as the teacher's pedagogical method. I think that this can be extended to mean that learning is greater and better when there is biorhythmical compatibility between student and teacher.

In his book *Teacher and Child*, Dr. Haim G. Ginott tells the parable of a house on fire. In a dark attic room a man is sleeping. The firemen try to save him with ladders but fail. Finally, the firechief says, "Wake him up, and he can save himself." Biorhythms should be the firechief awakening human being to ways to help themselves.

Yoshiyuki Okimura instituted a system of reports from mothers of children on whom biorhythm programs were being used. In one of them, a mother with two children said how happy she was at the courage and calm the knowledge of biorhythm had given her in dealing with her children. She had been awakened to ways to help her children and, in all likelihood, herself as well. This is why I insist that biorhythm is a science of timing and a science of tolerance and allowance.

Slump

This section offers reference material on how you can employ your knowledge of biorhythm from the standpoint of health design to recover from slump conditions brought on by chronic fatigue.

Slump—a prolonged period when a person is unable to perform as well as he usually can—almost invariably arises as a consequence of chronic fatigue. But it can act as autosuggestion on the mind of the individual and make it very difficult for him to break out of the slump condition. Sportsmen, especially veterans, usually have highly developed and sensitive motor nervous systems. This means that those nervous systems are delicate and susceptible to slump and the autosuggestion that causes it to persist. Of course, slump occurs in the lives of ordinary people as well. Executives are prone to it because of the stress involved in their work. Lower ranking company officers find that the tension created by pressure from the people below them and orders from their superiors generates fatigue and slump. Pressure exerted in Japan on young people to pass college entrance examinations frequently causes slump. In the cases of such students, as in those of middle-grade executives, failure to break out of the slump has been known to lead to suicide.

But it is possible to make a clear division between chronic fatigue and slump caused by hyperactivity of nervous suppressions, which make it impossible to snap out of the slump. Research on slump condition in fighter pilots during World War II showed that the state is produced by a loss of mental and physical positiveness. Conditioned reflexes reach a verveless state comparable to that of stale beer. This is true slump, which, objectively viewed, is a kind of neurosis, as the majority of psychiatrists would diagnose it.

Slump is of so many different kinds that treating it by occupation or cause is beyond the scope of this book. But I can mention two conditions that must be fulfilled if one is to snap out of the condition. Those conditions are sound sleep and observation of the three biorhythmic cycles. Unless these conditions are fulfilled, no matter how many others are satisfied, the condition will remain uncured.

To get the proper amount of the proper kind of sleep requires application of serious life prescriptions. But if the person can sleep well, a condition for escape from slump has been established. Psychiatrists sometimes fail to understand how to treat patients because they do not ensure the fulfillment of this condition.

From the standpoint of biorhythm study, the rhythm between activity and rest in the twenty-four-hour period is ten or twenty times more important a life prescription than the PSI theory. Consequently, simply skillfully manipulating the PSI theory is not the same thing as putting biorhythm to use in the optimum sense. I have already explained this in the basic text and I restate it now as an important consideration in recovering from slump.

When chronic fatigue settles into slump with pronounced psychological elements, adrenalin and noradrenalin, which are related to stress, are secreted in undue amounts into the blood. Since these hormones cause increased urination, the person becomes dehydrated and tends to drink more coffee or tea than usual. The caffeine in these beverages is a kind of alkaloid that excites the brain and prevents sound sleep. Theobromine intensifies the dehydration process—it is used as a diuretic—and creates violent thirsts. The vicious circle—stress urination, excitement, urination— supported by the drinking of coffee and tea makes it difficult to snap out of slump.

A simple change of scene may not be enough to help the person sleep soundly. But a week traveling for pleasure and staying in the right kind of hotels should solve the problem. The hotel must be in a quiet place, and you must not forget to take plugs for the ears. When you have found a hotel that meets the requirements, stay for two or three days.

Some people immediately resort to tranquilizers and sleeping pills, but this does not cure the slump and can lead to melancholia and even suicide. In place of such things, adopt the custom of the nightcap and have a small glass of hot wine or heated Japanese *saké* before retiring. Do not drink coffee, tea, cola beverages, or other soft drinks because they deaden the appetite and retard recovery from chronic fatigue. A small amount of cool water is much better.

Do not force yourself to eat if you have no appetite, for this can produce adverse effects. The best foods are easily digested eggs, cheese, yogurt, veal, liver, or bean curd. To this may be added a small amount of fruit or fresh vegetables. When adherence to this regimen has restored normal rhythm to daily life, it will be time to turn to the biorhythm PSI theory.

"Often school children are seriously affected by slump. I recall a case of a young girl whose teacher was very much surprised when her ordinarily good school performance fell sharply for a full week. I found out the girl's birth year, month, and day and plotted her biorhythm calendar. I learned that she was in a slump because all of her cycles were simultaneously in negative phases."

This example is cited by Yoshiyuki Okimura, who gives several others in a book that he and I coauthored on biorhythm and education. He then goes on to say that, though children lack the ability to control themselves and therefore live more under the control of natural conditions than adults, teaching them how to use their own biorhythm can enable them to overcome slump and to have self-confidence in school work. If one hears on the morning weather forecast that there will be rain in the afternoon, one does not worry, but takes an umbrella to work. Biorhythm is a science of timing that enables the human being to know how to be prepared and in this way to improve in school work and other aspects of daily life. One of the things biorhythm can do is help a person escape from slump. What Okimura says about biorhythm in the lives of children is applicable to the lives of adults as well. But adults can evolve a more sophisticated behavioral science because, armed with greater self-control than children, they can take advantage of many things like Zen, Yoga, and autogenic training.

Epilogue

Perhaps many of my readers are surprised at the extent and depth of the subject of biorhythm. But, since it is a human science, it is naturally complicated. The study of biological cycles and biorhythm are both sciences of timing; consequently, it is foolish to entertain the simple belief that positive is always good and negative always bad. These two aspects of the whole situation should be thought of in terms of the contrast between night and day.

Biorhythm is not a superstitious and fatalistic system for fortune telling. This mistaken idea gains no ground when biorhythm is handled by physicians—Fliess himself was a physician—but false interpretations have won some popularity because of the efforts of people who know nothing about biology or medicine.

Fortunately Dr. Schultz developed the autogenic system of using autosuggestion—under a physician's guidance—to cure patients of illnesses that are related to stress: high blood pressure and disorders of the stomach and intestines. Physicians who place total confidence in medicines and mechanical treatments tend to despise such things. But, even in America, a country where material things are consider all-important, doctors are employing psychoanalysis and other treatments that do not rely solely on physical medicine. After all, medicines are only aids; it is the patient himself who actually cures the sickness.

Autogenic training and biorhythm used properly elevate the individual's awareness of health and of the need for safety. This in turn can reduce both the number of ill people and the number of accidents accompanying the rapid spread of motorization in many parts of the world. Once the validity and usefulness of the biorhythm system has been proved, we must all look forward to developments of a technology for the sake of respect for life. In Japan and other places, this kind of technology is sadly wanting.

In my work in Japan with reduction of accidents in taxi companies and other similar organizations, I have already proved the validity of the biorhythm system. But my system is somewhat different from the older biorhythm, because it includes behavioral science. My system can be called neo-Fliessian or neobiorhythm. From the philosophical standpoint, on the basis of the concept of phenomenology, my system may be called *Biotakt*. Neobiorhythm is an example of successful docking of natural and humanistic sciences.

Neobiorhythm is divided into many stages. The kindergarten level is the classical biorhythm of Fliess, according to which one simply looks at the calendar and uses it as reference in the planning of daily life. The primary-school level is the stage in which the individual prepares his own calendar and attempts to understand its meaning. The middle-and high-school level is the stage at which attempts are made to apply biorhythm in self-control. The university level is the stage at which the individual tries to fuse principles and applications and advances into further studies. The beginner must realize the existence of all three levels.

It is true that there is an element of mathematical calculation in biorhythm for the sake of forecasting, but this is only an expedient. In other words, biorhythm stresses organic renovation instead of inorganic repetition. Rooted in behavioral science, the philosophical nature of biorhythm is that of neobiorhythm or *Biotakt*. In other words, it is a fusion of biology, psychology, and ethics. In graphic terms, the input is awareness. This produces the largely visual feedback of biorhythm conditions and memoranda and notation columns (awareness, in other words, short-term motivation, is part of autogenic training). This results in natural adjustment of action, which, after this screening, becomes the output or biofeedback.

Biorhythm Conditions

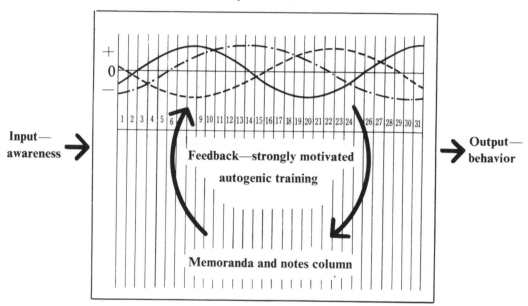

It is said that Mao Tse-tung always studied on the basis of experience and made science of the results. This is supposed to be the Chinese way. I remember vividly what Dr. Joseph Niedom, a professor at Cambridge and a specialist in the history of Chinese science, once said in a lecture. He claimed that the eight hundred million people of China are currently engaged in a vast experiment directed toward the creation of a society in which all persons can participate in all kinds of action. Behind the experiment are both ethics and moral conscience. He said that he foresees a resurrection of Confucianism because it strives to uncover the innate good in human beings. This, he believes, is an effort made in the hope of rediscovering human values. What he says is in complete agreement with my own feelings, except I see biorhythm as a way to elevate human values. Perhaps I feel this way because I am oriental.

As I have already pointed out, biorhythm application and study can be of great economical benefit. For instance, there are several bus companies and other transportation organizations in Japan that have used biorhythm training to set records for accident-free travel and in this way have saved money and improved the morale and physical and safety awareness of their personnel.

Maurice Chevalier voiced a sentiment in keeping with the teachings of biorhythm when he said that we must not merely endure our trials, but must put them to good use. When he visited the popular singer Mireille Mathieu in the hospital after she had suffered a serious injury in an automobile accident, he told her this and said that the English he had learned while in a German prisoner-of-war camp during World War I had helped him conquer the United States. Whether biorhythm can be of use to you depends on whether you agree with the Chinese in searching for human values, with Marurice Chevalier in his insistence that we must put our trials to use, and with me in agreeing with both of them.

Biorhythm can help in cultivating the following abilities, all of which are important and all too often missing in modern society.

(1) Calm as the outcome of cultivating self-control.
(2) Knack for planning things.
(3) Increased ability to cooperate with others.
(4) Habit of using things correctly.
(5) Skill and dexterity.

Tables

Biorhythms Calendar Table A (1873–1944)

year	P	S	I	year	P	S	I	year	P	S	I
1873	17	27	14	1897	14	25	26	1921	12	24	06
74	20	26	12	98	17	24	24	22	15	23	04
75	00	25	10	99	20	23	22	23	18	22	02
Month of Birth								Month of Birth			
JAN–FEB 76	03	24	08	1900	00	22	20	JAN–FEB 24	21	21	00
MAR–DEC ,,	02	23	07	Not a leap year				MAR–DEC ,,	20	20	32
1877	05	22	05	1901	03	21	18	1925	00	19	30
78	08	21	03	02	06	20	16	26	03	18	28
79	11	20	01	03	09	19	14	27	06	17	26
				Month of Birth							
JAN–FEB 80	14	19	32	JAN–FEB 04	12	18	12	JAN–FEB 28	09	16	24
MAR–DEC ,,	13	18	31	MAR–DEC ,,	11	17	11	MAR–DEC ,,	08	15	23
1881	16	17	29	1905	14	16	09	1929	11	14	21
82	19	16	27	06	17	15	07	30	14	13	19
83	22	15	25	07	20	14	05	31	17	12	17
JAN–FEB 84	02	14	23	JAN–FEB 08	00	13	03	JAN–FEB 32	20	11	15
MAR–DEC ,,	01	13	22	MAR–DEC ,,	22	12	02	MAR–DEC ,,	19	10	14
1885	04	12	20	1909	02	11	00	1933	22	09	12
86	07	11	18	10	05	10	31	34	02	08	10
87	10	10	16	11	08	09	29	35	05	07	08
JAN–FEB 88	13	09	14	JAN–FEB 12	11	08	27	JAN–FEB 36	08	06	06
MAR–DEC ,,	12	08	13	MAR–DEC ,,	10	07	26	MAR–DEC ,,	07	05	05
1889	15	07	11	1913	13	06	24	1937	10	04	03
90	18	06	09	14	16	05	22	38	13	03	01
91	·21	05	07	15	19	04	20	39	16	02	32
JAN–FEB 92	01	04	05	JAN–FEB 16	22	03	18	JAN–FEB 40	19	01	30
MAR–DEC ,,	00	03	04	MAR–DEC ,,	21	02	17	MAR–DEC ,,	18	00	29
1893	03	02	02	1917	01	01	15	1941	21	27	27
94	06	01	00	18	04	00	13	42	01	26	25
95	09	00	31	19	07	27	11	43	04	25	23
JAN–FEB 96	12	27	29	JAN–FEB 20	10	26	09	JAN–FEB 44	07	24	21
MAR–DEC ,,	11	26	28	MAR–DEC ,,	09	25	08	MAR–DEC ,,	06	23	20

Biorhythm Calendar Table A (1945–1916)

year	P	S	I	year	P	S	I	year	P	S	I
1945	09	22	18	**1969**	06	20	30	**1993**	03	18	09
46	12	21	16	**70**	09	19	28	**94**	06	17	07
47	15	20	14	**71**	12	18	26	**95**	09	16	05
Month of Birth				Month of Birth				Month of Birth			
JAN–FEB **48**	18	19	12	JAN–FEB **72**	15	17	24	JAN–FEB **96**	12	15	03
MAR–DEC ,,	17	18	11	MAR–DEC ,,	14	16	23	MAR–DEC ,,	11	14	02
1949	20	17	09	**1973**	17	15	21	**1997**	14	13	00
50	00	16	07	**74**	20	14	19	**98**	17	12	31
51	03	15	05	**75**	00	13	17	**99**	20	11	29
JAN–FEB **52**	06	14	03	JAN–FEB **76**	03	12	15	JAN–FEB **00**	00	10	27
MAR–DEC ,,	05	13	02	MAR–DEC ,,	02	11	14	MAR–DEC ,,	22	09	26
1953	08	12	00	**1977**	05	10	12	**2001**	02	08	24
54	11	11	31	**78**	08	09	10	**02**	05	07	22
55	14	10	29	**79**	11	08	08	**03**	08	06	20
JAN–FEB **56**	17	09	27	JAN–FEB **80**	14	07	06	JAN–FEB **04**	11	05	18
MAR–DEC ,,	16	08	26	MAR–DEC ,,	13	06	05	MAR–DEC ,,	10	04	17
1957	19	07	24	**1981**	16	05	03	**2005**	13	03	15
58	22	06	22	**82**	19	04	01	**06**	16	02	13
59	02	05	20	**83**	22	03	32	**07**	19	01	11
JAN–FEB **60**	05	04	18	JAN–FEB **84**	02	02	30	JAN–FEB **08**	22	00	09
MAR–DEC ,,	04	03	17	MAR–DEC ,,	01	01	29	MAR–DEC ,,	21	27	08
1961	07	02	15	**1985**	04	00	27	**2009**	01	26	06
62	10	01	13	**86**	07	27	25	**10**	04	25	04
63	13	00	11	**87**	10	26	23	**11**	07	24	02
JAN–FEB **64**	16	27	09	JAN–FEB **88**	13	25	21	JAN–FEB **12**	10	23	00
MAR–DEC ,,	15	26	08	MAR–DEC ,,	12	24	20	MAR–DEC ,,	09	22	32
1965	18	25	06	**1989**	15	23	18	**2013**	12	21	30
66	21	24	04	**90**	18	22	16	**14**	15	20	28
67	01	23	02	**91**	21	21	14	**15**	18	19	26
JAN–FEB **68**	04	22	00	JAN–FEB **92**	01	20	12	JAN–FEB **16**	21	18	24
MAR–DEC ,,	03	21	32	MAR–DEC ,,	00	19	11	MAR–DEC ,,	20	17	23

Biorhythm Calendar Table B (January–April)

Day	January P	S	I	February P	S	I	March P	S	I	April P	S	I
1	00	00	00	15	25	02	10	25	07	02	22	09
2	22	27	32	14	24	01	09	24	06	01	21	08
3	21	26	31	13	23	00	08	23	05	00	20	07
4	20	25	30	12	22	32	07	22	04	22	19	06
5	19	24	29	11	21	31	06	21	03	21	18	05
6	18	23	28	10	20	30	05	20	02	20	17	04
7	17	22	27	09	19	29	04	19	01	19	16	03
8	16	21	26	08	18	28	03	18	00	18	15	02
9	15	20	25	07	17	27	02	17	32	17	14	01
10	14	19	24	06	16	26	01	16	31	16	13	00
11	13	18	23	05	15	25	00	15	30	15	12	32
12	12	17	22	04	14	24	22	14	29	14	11	31
13	11	16	21	03	13	23	21	13	28	13	10	30
14	10	15	20	02	12	22	20	12	27	12	09	29
15	09	14	19	01	11	21	19	11	26	11	08	28
16	08	13	18	00	10	20	18	10	25	10	07	27
17	07	12	17	22	09	19	17	09	24	09	06	26
18	06	11	16	21	08	18	16	08	23	08	05	25
19	05	10	15	20	07	17	15	07	22	07	04	24
20	04	09	14	19	06	16	14	06	21	06	03	23
21	03	08	13	18	05	15	13	05	20	05	02	22
22	02	07	12	17	04	14	12	04	19	04	01	21
23	01	06	11	16	03	13	11	03	18	03	00	20
24	00	05	10	15	02	12	10	02	17	02	27	19
25	22	04	09	14	01	11	09	01	16	01	26	18
26	21	03	08	13	00	10	08	00	15	00	25	17
27	20	02	07	12	27	09	07	27	14	22	24	16
28	19	01	06	11	26	08	06	26	13	21	23	15
29	18	00	05	10	25	07	05	25	12	20	22	14
30	17	27	04				04	24	11	19	21	13
31	16	26	03				03	23	10			

Biorhythm Calendar Table B (May–August)

Day	May P	May S	May I	June P	June S	June I	July P	July S	July I	August P	August S	August I
1	18	20	12	10	17	14	03	15	17	18	12	19
2	17	19	11	09	16	13	02	14	16	17	11	18
3	16	18	10	08	15	12	01	13	15	16	10	17
4	15	17	09	07	14	11	00	12	14	15	09	16
5	14	16	08	06	13	10	22	11	13	14	08	15
6	13	15	07	05	12	09	21	10	12	13	07	14
7	12	14	06	04	11	08	20	09	11	12	06	13
8	11	13	05	03	10	07	19	08	10	11	05	12
9	10	12	04	02	09	06	18	07	09	10	04	11
10	09	11	03	01	08	05	17	06	08	09	03	10
11	08	10	02	00	07	04	16	05	07	08	02	09
12	07	09	01	22	06	03	15	04	06	07	01	08
13	06	08	00	21	05	02	14	03	05	06	00	07
14	05	07	32	20	04	01	13	02	04	05	27	06
15	04	06	31	19	03	00	12	01	03	04	26	05
16	03	05	30	18	02	32	11	00	02	03	25	04
17	02	04	29	17	01	31	10	27	01	02	24	03
18	01	03	28	16	00	30	09	26	00	01	23	02
19	00	02	27	15	27	29	08	25	32	00	22	01
20	22	01	26	14	26	28	07	24	31	22	21	00
21	21	00	25	13	25	27	06	23	30	21	20	32
22	20	27	24	12	24	26	05	22	29	20	19	31
23	19	26	23	11	23	25	04	21	28	19	18	30
24	18	25	22	10	22	24	03	20	27	18	17	29
25	17	24	21	09	21	23	02	19	26	17	16	28
26	16	23	20	08	20	22	01	18	25	16	15	27
27	15	22	19	07	19	21	00	17	24	15	14	26
28	14	21	18	06	18	20	22	16	23	14	13	25
29	13	20	17	05	17	19	21	15	22	13	12	24
30	12	19	16	04	16	18	20	14	21	12	11	23
31	11	18	15				19	13	20	11	10	22

Biorhythm Calendar Table B (September–December)

Day	September P	S	I	October P	S	I	November P	S	I	December P	S	I
1	10	09	21	03	07	24	18	04	26	11	02	29
2	09	08	20	02	06	23	17	03	25	10	01	28
3	08	07	19	01	05	22	16	02	24	09	00	27
4	07	06	18	00	04	21	15	01	23	08	27	26
5	06	05	17	22	03	20	14	00	22	07	26	25
6	05	04	16	21	02	19	13	27	21	06	25	24
7	04	03	15	20	01	18	12	26	20	05	24	23
8	03	02	14	19	00	17	11	25	19	04	23	22
9	02	01	13	18	27	16	10	24	18	03	22	21
10	01	00	12	17	26	15	09	23	17	02	21	20
11	00	27	11	16	25	14	08	22	16	01	20	19
12	22	26	10	15	24	13	07	21	15	00	19	18
13	21	25	09	14	23	12	06	20	14	22	18	17
14	20	24	08	13	22	11	05	19	13	21	17	16
15	19	23	07	12	21	10	04	18	12	20	16	15
16	18	22	06	11	20	09	03	17	11	19	15	14
17	17	21	05	10	19	08	02	16	10	18	14	13
18	16	20	04	09	18	07	01	15	09	17	13	12
19	15	19	03	08	17	06	00	14	08	16	12	11
20	14	18	02	07	16	05	22	13	07	15	11	10
21	13	17	01	06	15	04	21	12	06	14	10	09
22	12	16	00	05	14	03	20	11	05	13	09	08
23	11	15	32	04	13	02	19	10	04	12	08	07
24	10	14	31	03	12	01	18	09	03	11	07	06
25	09	13	30	02	11	00	17	08	02	10	06	05
26	08	12	29	01	10	32	16	07	01	09	05	04
27	07	11	28	00	09	31	15	06	00	08	04	03
28	06	10	27	22	08	30	14	05	32	07	03	02
29	05	09	26	21	07	29	13	04	31	06	02	01
30	04	08	25	20	06	28	12	03	30	05	01	00
31				19	05	27				04	00	32

Biorhythm Calendar Table C (1961–1968)

Month	1961 P	S	I	1962 P	S	I	1963 P	S	I	1964 P	S	I
1	16	26	18	13	27	20	10	00	22	07	01	24
2	01	01	16	21	03	18	18	03	20	15	04	22
3	06	01	11	03	02	13	00	03	15	21	05	18
4	14	04	09	11	05	11	08	06	13	06	08	16
5	21	06	06	18	07	08	15	08	10	13	10	13
6	06	09	04	03	10	06	00	11	08	21	13	11
7	13	11	01	10	12	03	07	13	05	05	15	08
8	21	14	32	18	15	01	15	16	03	13	18	06
9	06	17	30	03	18	32	00	19	01	21	21	04
10	13	19	27	10	20	29	07	21	31	05	23	01
11	21	22	25	18	23	27	15	24	29	13	26	32
12	05	24	22	02	25	24	22	26	26	20	00	29

Month	1965 P	S	I	1966 P	S	I	1967 P	S	I	1968 P	S	I
1	05	03	27	02	04	29	22	05	31	19	06	00
2	13	06	25	10	07	27	07	08	29	04	09	31
3	18	06	20	15	07	22	12	08	24	10	10	27
4	03	09	18	00	10	20	20	11	22	18	13	25
5	10	11	15	07	12	17	04	13	19	02	15	22
6	18	14	13	15	15	15	12	16	17	10	18	20
7	02	16	10	22	17	12	19	18	14	17	20	17
8	10	19	08	07	20	10	04	21	12	02	23	15
9	18	22	06	15	23	08	12	24	10	10	26	13
10	02	24	03	22	25	05	19	26	07	17	00	10
11	10	27	01	07	00	03	04	01	05	02	03	08
12	17	01	31	14	02	00	11	03	02	09	05	05

Biorhythm Calendar Table C (1969–1976)

Month	1969			1970			1971			1972		
	P	S	I	P	S	I	P	S	I	P	S	I
1	17	08	03	14	09	05	11	10	07	08	11	09
2	02	11	01	22	12	03	19	13	05	16	14	07
3	07	11	29	14	12	31	01	13	00	22	15	03
4	15	14	27	12	15	29	09	16	31	07	18	01
5	22	16	24	19	17	26	16	18	28	14	20	31
6	07	19	22	04	20	24	01	21	26	22	23	29
7	14	21	19	11	22	21	08	23	23	06	25	26
8	22	24	17	19	25	19	16	26	21	14	00	24
9	07	27	15	04	00	17	01	01	19	22	03	22
10	14	01	12	11	02	14	08	03	16	06	05	19
11	22	04	10	19	05	12	16	06	14	14	08	17
12	06	06	07	03	07	09	00	08	11	21	10	14

Month	1973			1974			1975			1976		
	P	S	I	P	S	I	P	S	I	P	S	I
1	06	13	12	03	14	14	00	15	16	20	16	18
2	14	16	10	11	17	12	08	18	14	05	19	16
3	19	16	05	16	17	07	13	18	09	11	20	12
4	04	19	03	01	20	05	21	21	07	19	23	10
5	11	21	00	08	22	02	05	23	04	03	25	07
6	19	24	31	16	25	00	13	26	02	11	00	05
7	03	26	28	00	27	30	20	00	32	18	02	02
8	11	01	26	08	02	28	05	03	30	03	05	00
9	19	04	24	16	05	26	13	06	28	11	08	31
10	03	06	21	00	07	23	20	08	25	18	10	28
11	11	09	19	08	10	21	05	11	23	03	13	26
12	18	11	16	15	12	18	12	13	20	10	15	23

Biorhythm Calendar Table C (1977–1984)

Month	1977 P	S	I	1978 P	S	I	1979 P	S	I	1980 P	S	I
1	18	18	21	15	19	23	12	20	25	09	21	27
2	03	21	19	00	22	21	20	23	23	17	24	25
3	18	21	14	05	22	16	02	23	18	00	25	21
4	16	24	12	13	25	14	10	26	16	08	00	19
5	00	26	09	20	27	11	17	00	13	15	02	16
6	08	01	07	05	02	09	02	03	11	00	05	14
7	15	03	04	12	04	06	09	05	08	07	07	11
8	00	06	02	20	07	04	17	08	06	15	10	09
9	08	09	00	05	10	02	02	11	04	00	13	07
10	15	11	30	12	12	32	09	13	01	07	15	04
11	00	14	28	20	15	30	17	16	32	15	18	02
12	07	16	25	04	17	27	01	18	29	22	20	32

Month	1981 P	S	I	1982 P	S	I	1983 P	S	I	1984 P	S	I
1	07	23	30	04	24	32	01	25	01	21	26	03
2	15	26	28	12	27	30	09	00	32	06	01	01
3	20	26	23	17	27	25	14	00	27	12	02	30
4	05	01	21	02	02	23	22	03	25	20	05	28
5	12	03	18	09	04	20	06	05	22	04	07	25
6	20	06	16	17	07	18	14	08	20	12	10	23
7	04	08	13	01	09	15	21	10	17	19	12	20
8	12	11	11	09	12	13	06	13	15	04	15	18
9	20	14	09	17	15	11	14	16	13	12	18	16
10	04	16	06	01	17	08	21	18	10	19	20	13
11	12	19	04	09	20	06	06	21	08	04	23	11
12	19	21	01	16	22	03	13	23	05	11	25	08

Biorhythm Calendar Table C (1985–1992)

Month	1985 P	S	I	1986 P	S	I	1987 P	S	I	1988 P	S	I
1	19	00	06	16	01	08	13	02	10	10	03	12
2	04	03	04	01	04	06	21	05	08	18	06	10
3	09	03	32	06	04	01	03	05	03	01	07	06
4	17	06	30	14	07	32	11	08	01	09	10	04
5	01	08	27	21	09	29	18	10	31	16	12	01
6	09	11	25	06	12	27	03	13	29	01	15	32
7	16	13	22	13	14	24	10	15	26	08	17	29
8	01	16	20	21	17	22	18	18	24	16	20	27
9	09	19	18	06	20	20	03	21	22	01	23	25
10	16	21	15	13	22	17	10	23	19	08	25	22
11	01	24	13	21	25	15	18	26	17	16	00	20
12	08	26	10	05	27	12	02	00	14	00	02	17

Month	1989 P	S	I	1990 P	S	I	1991 P	S	I	1992 P	S	I
1	08	05	15	05	06	17	02	07	19	22	08	21
2	16	08	13	13	09	15	10	10	17	07	11	19
3	21	08	08	18	09	10	15	10	12	13	12	15
4	06	11	06	03	12	08	00	13	10	21	15	13
5	13	13	03	10	14	05	07	15	07	05	17	10
6	21	16	01	18	17	03	15	18	05	13	20	08
7	05	18	31	02	19	00	22	20	02	20	22	05
8	13	21	29	10	22	31	07	23	00	05	25	03
9	21	24	27	18	25	29	15	26	31	13	00	01
10	05	26	24	02	27	26	22	00	28	20	02	31
11	13	01	22	10	02	24	07	03	26	05	05	29
12	20	03	19	17	04	21	14	05	23	12	07	26

Biorhythm Calendar Table C (1993–2000)

Month	1993			1994			1995			1996		
	P	S	I	P	S	I	P	S	I	P	S	I
1	20	10	24	17	11	26	14	12	28	11	13	30
2	05	13	22	02	14	24	22	15	26	19	16	28
3	10	13	17	07	14	19	04	15	21	02	17	24
4	18	16	15	15	17	17	12	18	19	10	20	22
5	02	18	12	22	19	14	19	20	16	17	22	19
6	10	21	10	07	22	12	04	23	14	02	25	17
7	17	23	07	14	24	09	11	25	11	09	27	14
8	02	26	05	22	27	07	19	00	09	17	02	12
9	10	01	03	07	02	05	04	03	07	02	05	10
10	17	03	00	14	04	02	11	05	04	09	07	07
11	02	06	31	22	07	00	19	08	02	17	10	05
12	09	08	28	06	09	30	03	10	32	01	12	02

Month	1997			1998			1999			2000		
	P	S	I	P	S	I	P	S	I	P	S	I
1	09	15	00	06	16	02	03	17	04	00	18	06
2	17	18	31	14	19	00	11	20	02	08	21	04
3	22	18	26	19	19	28	16	20	30	14	22	00
4	07	21	24	04	22	26	01	23	28	22	25	31
5	14	23	21	11	24	23	08	25	25	06	27	28
6	22	26	19	19	27	21	16	00	23	14	02	26
7	06	00	16	03	01	18	00	02	20	21	04	23
8	14	03	14	11	04	16	08	05	18	06	07	21
9	22	06	12	19	07	14	16	08	16	14	10	19
10	06	08	09	03	09	11	00	10	13	21	12	16
11	14	11	07	11	12	09	08	13	11	06	15	14
12	21	13	04	18	14	06	15	15	08	13	17	11

Biorhythm Calendar Table C (2001–2008)

Month	2001 P	S	I	2002 P	S	I	2003 P	S	I	2004 P	S	I
1	21	20	09	18	21	11	15	22	13	12	23	15
2	06	23	07	03	24	09	00	25	11	20	26	13
3	11	23	02	08	24	04	05	25	06	03	27	09
4	19	26	00	16	27	02	13	00	04	11	02	07
5	03	00	30	00	01	32	20	02	01	18	04	04
6	11	03	28	08	04	30	05	05	32	03	07	02
7	18	05	25	15	06	27	12	07	29	10	09	32
8	03	08	23	00	09	25	20	10	27	18	12	30
9	11	11	21	08	12	23	05	13	25	03	15	28
10	18	13	18	15	14	20	12	15	22	10	17	25
11	03	16	16	00	17	18	20	18	20	18	20	23
12	10	18	13	07	19	15	04	20	17	02	22	20

Month	2005 P	S	I	2006 P	S	I	2007 P	S	I	2008 P	S	I
1	10	25	18	07	26	20	04	27	22	01	00	24
2	18	00	16	15	01	18	12	02	20	09	03	22
3	00	00	11	20	01	13	17	02	15	15	04	18
4	08	03	09	05	04	11	02	05	13	00	07	16
5	15	05	06	12	06	08	09	07	10	07	09	13
6	00	08	04	20	09	06	17	10	08	15	12	11
7	07	10	01	04	11	03	01	12	05	22	14	08
8	15	13	32	12	14	01	09	15	03	07	17	06
9	00	16	30	20	17	32	17	18	01	15	20	04
10	07	18	27	04	19	29	01	20	31	22	22	01
11	15	21	25	12	22	27	09	23	29	07	25	32
12	22	23	22	19	24	24	16	25	26	14	27	29

Biorhythm Calendar Table C (2009–2016)

Month	2009			2010			2011			2012		
	P	S	I	P	S	I	P	S	I	P	S	I
1	22	02	27	19	03	29	16	04	31	13	05	00
2	07	05	25	04	06	27	01	07	29	21	08	31
3	12	05	20	09	06	22	06	07	24	04	09	27
4	20	08	18	17	09	20	14	10	22	12	12	25
5	04	10	15	01	11	17	21	12	19	19	14	22
6	12	13	13	09	14	15	06	15	17	04	17	20
7	19	15	10	16	16	12	13	17	14	11	19	17
8	04	18	08	01	19	10	21	20	12	19	22	15
9	12	21	06	09	22	08	06	23	10	04	25	13
10	19	23	03	16	24	05	13	25	07	11	27	10
11	04	26	01	01	27	03	21	00	05	19	02	08
12	11	00	31	08	01	00	05	02	02	03	04	05

Month	2013			2014			2015			2016		
	P	S	I	P	S	I	P	S	I	P	S	I
1	11	07	03	08	08	05	05	09	07	02	10	09
2	19	10	01	16	11	03	13	12	05	10	13	07
3	01	10	29	21	11	31	18	12	00	16	14	03
4	09	13	27	06	14	29	03	15	31	01	17	01
5	16	15	24	13	16	26	10	17	28	08	19	31
6	01	18	22	21	19	24	18	20	26	16	22	29
7	08	20	19	05	21	21	02	22	23	00	24	26
8	16	23	17	13	24	19	10	25	21	08	27	24
9	01	26	15	21	27	17	18	00	19	16	02	22
10	08	00	12	05	01	14	02	02	16	00	04	19
11	16	03	10	13	04	12	10	05	14	08	07	17
12	00	05	07	20	06	09	17	07	11	15	09	14

Tatai Table A (1881–1952)

year	P	S	I	year	P	S	I	year	P	S	I
1881	09	13	06	1905	11	14	26	1929	14	16	14
82	06	14	08	06	08	15	28	30	11	17	16
83	03	15	10	07	05	16	30	31	08	18	18
Month of Birth				Month of Birth				Month of Birth			
JAN–FEB 84	00	16	12	JAN–FEB 08	02	17	32	JAN–FEB 32	05	19	20
MAR–DEC ,,	01	17	13	MAR–DEC ,,	03	18	00	MAR–DEC ,,	06	20	21
1885	21	18	15	1909	00	19	02	1933	03	21	23
86	18	19	17	10	20	20	04	34	00	22	25
87	15	20	19	11	17	21	06	35	20	23	27
JAN–FEB 88	12	21	21	JAN–FEB 12	14	22	08	JAN–FEB 36	17	24	29
MAR–DEC ,,	13	22	22	MAR–DEC ,,	15	23	09	MAR–DEC ,,	18	25	30
1889	10	23	24	1913	12	24	11	1937	15	26	32
90	07	24	26	14	09	25	13	38	12	27	01
91	04	25	28	15	06	26	15	39	09	00	03
JAN–FEB 92	01	26	30	JAN–FEB 16	03	27	17	JAN–FEB 40	06	01	05
MAR–DEC ,,	02	27	31	MAR–DEC ,,	04	00	18	MAR–DEC ,,	07	02	06
1893	22	00	00	1917	01	01	20	1941	04	03	08
94	19	01	02	18	21	02	22	42	01	04	10
95	16	02	04	19	18	03	24	43	21	05	12
JAN–FEB 96	13	03	06	JAN–FEB 20	15	04	26	JAN–FEB 44	18	06	14
MAR–DEC ,,	14	04	07	MAR–DEC ,,	16	05	27	MAR–DEC ,,	19	07	15
1897	11	05	09	1921	13	06	29	1945	16	08	17
98	08	06	11	22	10	07	31	46	13	09	19
99	05	07	13	23	07	08	00	47	10	10	21
1900	02	08	15	JAN–FEB 24	04	09	02	JAN–FEB 48	07	11	23
Not a leap year				MAR–DEC ,,	05	10	03	MAR–DEC ,,	08	12	24
1901	22	09	17	1925	02	11	05	1949	05	13	26
02	19	10	19	26	22	12	07	50	02	14	28
03	16	11	21	27	19	13	09	51	22	15	30
JAN–FEB 04	13	12	23	JAN–FEB 28	16	14	11	JAN–FEB 52	19	16	32
MAR–DEC ,,	14	13	24	MAR–DEC ,,	17	15	12	MAR–DEC ,,	20	17	00

Tatai Table A (1953–2024)

year	P	S	I	year	P	S	I	year	P	S	I
1953	17	18	02	**1977**	20	20	23	**2001**	00	22	11
54	14	19	04	**78**	17	21	25	**02**	20	23	13
55	11	20	06	**79**	14	22	27	**03**	17	24	15
Month of Birth				Month of Birth				Month of Birth			
JAN–FEB **56**	08	21	08	JAN–FEB **80**	11	23	29	JAN–FEB **04**	14	25	17
MAR–DEC ,,	09	22	09	MAR–DEC ,,	12	24	30	MAR–DEC ,,	15	26	18
1957	06	23	11	**1981**	09	25	32	**2005**	12	27	20
58	03	24	13	**82**	06	26	01	**06**	09	00	22
59	00	25	15	**83**	03	27	03	**07**	06	01	24
JAN–FEB **60**	20	26	17	JAN–FEB **84**	00	00	05	JAN–FEB **08**	03	02	26
MAR–DEC ,,	21	27	18	MAR–DEC ,,	01	01	06	MAR–DEC ,,	04	03	27
1961	18	00	20	**1985**	21	02	08	**2009**	01	04	29
62	15	01	22	**86**	18	03	10	**10**	21	05	31
63	12	02	24	**87**	15	04	12	**11**	18	06	00
JAN–FEB **64**	09	03	26	JAN–FEB **88**	12	05	14	JAN–FEB **12**	15	07	02
MAR–DEC ,,	10	04	27	MAR–DEC ,,	13	06	15	MAR–DEC ,,	16	08	03
1965	07	05	29	**1989**	10	07	17	**2013**	13	09	05
66	04	06	31	**90**	07	08	19	**14**	10	10	07
67	01	07	00	**91**	04	09	21	**15**	07	11	09
JAN–FEB **68**	21	08	02	JAN–FEB **92**	01	10	23	JAN–FEB **16**	04	12	11
MAR–DEC ,,	22	09	03	MAR–DEC ,,	02	11	24	MAR–DEC ,,	05	13	12
1969	19	10	05	**1993**	22	12	26	**2017**	02	14	14
70	16	11	07	**94**	19	13	28	**18**	22	15	16
71	13	12	09	**95**	16	14	30	**19**	19	16	18
JAN–FEB **72**	10	13	11	JAN–FEB **96**	13	15	32	JAN–FEB **20**	16	17	20
MAR–DEC ,,	11	14	12	MAR–DEC ,,	14	16	00	MAR–DEC ,,	17	18	21
1973	08	15	14	**1997**	11	17	02	**2021**	14	19	23
74	05	16	16	**98**	08	18	04	**22**	11	20	25
75	02	17	18	**99**	05	19	06	**23**	08	21	27
JAN–FEB **76**	22	18	20	JAN–FEB **2000**	02	20	08	JAN–FEB **24**	05	22	29
MAR–DEC ,,	00	19	21	MAR–DEC ,,	03	21	09	MAR–DEC ,,	06	23	30

Tatai Table B (January–April)

day	January			February			March			April		
	P	S	I	P	S	I	P	S	I	P	S	I
1	22	27	32	07	02	30	12	02	25	20	05	23
2	00	00	00	08	03	31	13	03	26	21	06	24
3	01	01	01	09	04	32	14	04	27	22	07	25
4	02	02	02	10	05	00	15	05	28	00	08	26
5	03	03	03	11	06	01	16	06	29	01	09	27
6	04	04	04	12	07	02	17	07	30	02	10	28
7	05	05	05	13	08	03	18	08	31	03	11	29
8	06	06	06	14	09	04	19	09	32	04	12	30
9	07	07	07	15	10	05	20	10	00	05	13	31
10	08	08	08	16	11	06	21	11	01	06	14	32
11	09	09	09	17	12	07	22	12	02	07	15	00
12	10	10	10	18	13	08	00	13	03	08	16	01
13	11	11	11	19	14	09	01	14	04	09	17	02
14	12	12	12	20	15	10	02	15	05	10	18	03
15	13	13	13	21	16	11	03	16	06	11	19	04
16	14	14	14	22	17	12	04	17	07	12	20	05
17	15	15	15	00	18	13	05	18	08	13	21	06
18	16	16	16	01	19	14	06	19	09	14	22	07
19	17	17	17	02	20	15	07	20	10	15	23	08
20	18	18	18	03	21	16	08	21	11	16	24	09
21	19	19	19	04	22	17	09	22	12	17	25	10
22	20	20	20	05	23	18	10	23	13	18	26	11
23	21	21	21	06	24	19	11	24	14	19	27	12
24	22	22	22	07	25	20	12	25	15	20	00	13
25	00	23	23	08	26	21	13	26	16	21	01	14
26	01	24	24	09	27	22	14	27	17	22	02	15
27	02	25	25	10	00	23	15	00	18	00	03	16
28	03	26	26	11	01	24	16	01	19	01	04	17
29	04	27	27	12	02	25	17	02	20	02	05	18
30	05	00	28				18	03	21	03	06	19
31	06	01	29				19	04	22			

Tatai Table B (May–August)

Day	May			June			July			August		
	P	S	I	P	S	I	P	S	I	P	S	I
1	04	07	20	12	10	18	19	12	15	04	15	13
2	05	08	21	13	11	19	20	13	16	05	16	14
3	06	09	22	14	12	20	21	14	17	06	17	15
4	07	10	23	15	13	21	22	15	18	07	18	16
5	08	11	24	16	14	22	00	16	19	08	19	17
6	09	12	25	17	15	23	01	17	20	09	20	18
7	10	13	26	18	16	24	02	18	21	10	21	19
8	11	14	27	19	17	25	03	19	22	11	22	20
9	12	15	28	20	18	26	04	20	23	12	23	21
10	13	16	29	21	19	27	05	21	24	13	24	22
11	14	17	30	22	20	28	06	22	25	14	25	23
12	15	18	31	00	21	29	07	23	26	15	26	24
13	16	19	32	01	22	30	08	24	27	16	27	25
14	17	20	00	02	23	31	09	25	28	17	00	26
15	18	21	01	03	24	32	10	26	29	18	01	27
16	19	22	02	04	25	00	11	27	30	19	02	28
17	20	23	03	05	26	01	12	00	31	20	03	29
18	21	24	04	06	27	02	13	01	32	21	04	30
19	22	25	05	07	00	03	14	02	00	22	05	31
20	00	26	06	08	01	04	15	03	01	00	06	32
21	01	27	07	09	02	05	16	04	02	01	07	00
22	02	00	08	10	03	06	17	05	03	02	08	01
23	03	01	09	11	04	07	18	06	04	03	09	02
24	04	02	10	12	05	08	19	07	05	04	10	03
25	05	03	11	13	06	09	20	08	06	05	11	04
26	06	04	12	14	07	10	21	09	07	06	12	05
27	07	05	13	15	08	11	22	10	08	07	13	06
28	08	06	14	16	09	12	00	11	09	08	14	07
29	09	07	15	17	10	13	01	12	10	09	15	08
30	10	08	16	18	11	14	02	13	11	10	16	09
31	11	09	17				03	14	12	11	17	10

Tatai Table B (September–December)

Day	September			October			November			December		
	P	S	I	P	S	I	P	S	I	P	S	I
1	12	18	11	19	20	08	04	23	06	11	25	03
2	13	19	12	20	21	09	05	24	07	12	26	04
3	14	20	13	21	22	10	06	25	08	13	27	05
4	15	21	14	22	23	11	07	26	09	14	00	06
5	16	22	15	00	24	12	08	27	10	15	01	07
6	17	23	16	01	25	13	09	00	11	16	02	08
7	18	24	17	02	26	14	10	01	12	17	03	09
8	19	25	18	03	27	15	11	02	13	18	04	10
9	20	26	19	04	00	16	12	03	14	19	05	11
10	21	27	20	05	01	17	13	04	15	20	06	12
11	22	00	21	06	02	18	14	05	16	21	07	13
12	00	01	22	07	03	19	15	06	17	22	08	14
13	01	02	23	08	04	20	16	07	18	00	09	15
14	02	03	24	09	05	21	17	08	19	01	10	16
15	03	04	25	10	06	22	18	09	20	02	11	17
16	04	05	26	11	07	23	19	10	21	03	12	18
17	05	06	27	12	08	24	20	11	22	04	13	19
18	06	07	28	13	09	25	21	12	23	05	14	20
19	07	08	29	14	10	26	22	13	24	06	15	21
20	08	09	30	15	11	27	00	14	25	07	16	22
21	09	10	31	16	12	28	01	15	26	08	17	23
22	10	11	32	17	13	29	02	16	27	09	18	24
23	11	12	00	18	14	30	03	17	28	10	19	25
24	12	13	01	19	15	31	04	18	29	11	20	26
25	13	14	02	20	16	32	05	19	30	12	21	27
26	14	15	03	21	17	00	06	20	31	13	22	28
27	15	16	04	22	18	01	07	21	32	14	23	29
28	16	17	05	00	19	02	08	22	00	15	24	30
29	17	18	06	01	20	03	09	23	01	16	25	31
39	18	19	07	02	21	04	10	24	02	17	26	32
31				03	22	05				18	27	00

Tatai Table C (1945–1952)

Month	1945			1946			1947			1948		
	P	S	I	P	S	I	P	S	I	P	S	I
1	09	22	18	12	21	16	15	20	14	18	19	12
2	01	19	20	04	18	18	07	17	16	10	16	14
3	19	19	25	22	18	23	02	17	21	04	15	18
4	11	16	27	14	15	25	17	14	23	19	12	20
5	04	14	30	07	13	28	10	12	26	12	10	23
6	19	11	32	22	10	30	02	09	28	04	07	25
7	12	09	02	15	08	00	18	07	31	20	05	28
8	04	06	04	07	05	02	10	04	00	12	02	30
9	19	03	06	22	02	04	02	01	02	04	27	32
10	12	01	09	15	00	07	18	27	05	20	25	02
11	04	26	11	07	25	09	10	24	07	12	22	04
12	20	24	14	00	23	12	03	22	10	05	20	07

Month	1949			1950			1951			1952		
	P	S	I	P	S	I	P	S	I	P	S	I
1	20	17	09	00	16	07	03	15	05	06	14	03
2	12	14	11	15	13	09	18	12	07	21	11	05
3	07	14	16	10	13	14	13	12	12	15	10	09
4	22	11	18	02	10	16	05	09	14	07	07	11
5	15	09	21	18	08	19	21	07	17	00	05	14
6	07	06	23	10	05	21	13	04	19	15	02	16
7	00	04	26	03	03	24	06	02	22	08	00	19
8	15	01	28	18	00	26	21	27	24	00	25	21
9	07	26	30	10	25	28	13	24	26	15	22	23
10	00	24	00	03	23	31	06	22	29	08	20	26
11	15	21	02	18	20	00	21	19	31	00	17	28
12	08	19	05	11	18	03	14	17	01	16	15	31

Tatai Table C (1953–1960)

Month	1953 P	S	I	1954 P	S	I	1955 P	S	I	1956 P	S	I
1	08	12	00	11	11	31	14	10	29	17	09	27
2	00	09	02	03	08	00	06	07	31	09	06	29
3	18	09	07	21	08	05	01	07	03	03	05	00
4	10	06	09	13	05	07	16	04	05	18	02	02
5	03	04	12	06	03	10	09	02	08	11	00	05
6	18	01	14	21	00	12	01	27	10	03	25	07
7	11	27	17	14	26	15	17	25	13	19	23	10
8	03	24	19	06	23	17	09	22	15	11	20	12
9	18	21	21	21	20	19	01	19	17	03	17	14
10	11	19	24	14	18	22	17	17	20	19	15	17
11	03	16	26	06	15	24	09	14	22	11	12	19
12	19	14	29	22	13	27	02	12	25	04	10	22

Month	1957 P	S	I	1958 P	S	I	1959 P	S	I	1960 P	S	I
1	19	07	24	22	06	22	02	05	20	05	04	18
2	11	04	26	14	03	24	17	02	22	20	01	20
3	06	04	31	09	03	29	12	02	27	14	00	24
4	21	01	00	01	00	31	04	27	29	06	25	26
5	14	27	03	17	26	01	20	25	32	22	23	29
6	06	24	05	09	23	03	12	22	01	14	20	31
7	22	22	08	02	21	06	05	20	04	07	18	01
8	14	19	10	17	18	08	20	17	06	22	15	03
9	06	16	12	09	15	10	12	14	08	14	12	05
10	22	14	15	02	13	13	05	12	11	07	10	08
11	14	11	17	17	10	15	20	09	13	22	07	10
12	07	09	20	10	08	18	13	07	16	15	05	13

Tatai Table C (1961–1968)

Month	1961 P	S	I	1962 P	S	I	1963 P	S	I	1964 P	S	I
1	07	02	15	10	01	13	13	00	11	16	27	09
2	22	27	17	02	26	15	05	25	13	08	24	11
3	17	27	22	20	26	20	00	25	18	02	23	15
4	09	24	24	12	23	22	15	22	20	17	20	17
5	02	22	27	05	21	25	08	20	23	10	18	20
6	17	19	29	20	18	27	00	17	25	02	15	22
7	10	17	32	13	16	30	16	15	28	18	13	25
8	02	14	01	05	13	32	08	12	30	10	10	27
9	17	11	03	20	10	01	00	09	32	02	07	29
10	10	09	06	13	08	04	16	07	02	18	05	32
11	02	06	08	05	05	06	08	04	04	10	02	01
12	18	04	11	21	03	09	01	02	07	03	00	04

Month	1965 P	S	I	1966 P	S	I	1967 P	S	I	1968 P	S	I
1	18	25	06	21	24	04	01	23	02	04	22	00
2	10	22	08	13	21	06	16	20	04	19	19	02
3	05	22	13	08	21	11	11	20	09	13	18	06
4	20	19	15	00	18	13	03	17	11	05	15	08
5	13	17	18	16	16	16	19	15	14	21	13	11
6	05	14	20	08	13	18	11	12	16	13	10	13
7	21	12	23	01	11	21	04	10	19	06	08	16
8	13	09	25	16	08	23	19	07	21	21	05	18
9	05	06	27	08	05	25	11	04	23	13	02	20
10	21	04	30	01	03	28	04	02	26	06	00	23
11	13	01	32	16	00	30	19	27	28	21	25	25
12	06	27	02	09	26	00	12	25	31	14	23	28

Tatai Table C (1969–1976)

Month	1969 P	S	I	1970 P	S	I	1971 P	S	I	1972 P	S	I
1	06	20	30	09	19	28	12	18	26	15	17	24
2	21	17	32	01	16	30	04	15	28	07	14	26
3	16	17	04	19	16	02	22	15	00	01	13	30
4	08	14	06	11	13	04	14	12	02	16	10	32
5	01	12	09	04	11	07	07	10	05	09	08	02
6	16	09	11	19	08	09	22	07	07	01	05	04
7	09	07	14	12	06	12	15	05	10	17	03	07
8	01	04	16	04	03	14	07	02	12	09	00	09
9	16	01	18	19	00	16	22	27	14	01	25	11
10	09	27	21	12	26	19	15	25	17	17	23	14
11	01	24	23	04	23	21	07	22	19	09	20	16
12	17	22	26	20	21	24	00	20	22	02	18	19

Month	1973 P	S	I	1974 P	S	I	1975 P	S	I	1976 P	S	I
1	17	15	21	20	14	19	00	13	17	03	12	15
2	09	12	23	12	11	21	15	10	19	18	09	17
3	04	12	28	07	11	26	10	10	24	12	08	21
4	19	09	30	22	08	28	02	07	26	04	05	23
5	12	07	00	15	06	31	18	05	29	20	03	26
6	04	04	02	07	03	00	10	02	31	12	00	28
7	20	02	05	00	01	03	03	00	01	05	26	31
8	12	27	07	15	26	05	18	25	03	20	23	00
9	04	24	09	07	23	07	10	22	05	12	20	02
10	20	22	12	00	21	10	03	20	08	05	18	05
11	12	19	14	15	18	12	18	17	10	20	15	07
12	05	17	17	08	16	15	11	15	13	13	13	10

Tatai Table C (1977–1984)

Month	1977			1978			1979			1980		
	P	S	I	P	S	I	P	S	I	P	S	I
1	05	10	12	08	09	10	11	08	08	14	07	06
2	20	07	14	00	06	12	03	05	10	06	04	08
3	15	07	19	18	06	17	21	05	15	00	03	12
4	07	04	21	10	03	19	13	02	17	15	00	14
5	00	02	24	03	01	22	06	00	20	08	26	17
6	15	27	26	18	26	24	21	25	22	00	23	19
7	08	25	29	11	24	27	14	23	25	16	21	22
8	00	22	31	03	21	29	06	20	27	08	18	24
9	15	19	00	18	18	31	21	17	29	00	15	26
10	08	17	03	11	16	01	14	15	32	16	13	29
11	00	14	05	03	13	03	06	12	01	08	10	31
12	16	12	08	19	11	06	22	10	04	01	08	01

Month	1981			1982			1983			1984		
	P	S	I	P	S	I	P	S	I	P	S	I
1	16	05	03	19	04	01	22	03	32	02	02	30
2	08	02	05	11	01	03	14	00	01	17	27	32
3	03	02	10	06	01	08	09	00	06	11	26	03
4	18	27	12	21	26	10	01	25	08	03	23	05
5	11	25	15	14	24	13	17	23	11	19	21	08
6	03	22	17	06	21	15	09	20	13	11	18	10
7	19	20	20	22	19	18	02	18	16	04	16	13
8	11	17	22	14	16	20	17	15	18	19	13	15
9	03	14	24	06	13	22	09	12	20	11	10	17
10	19	12	27	22	11	25	02	10	23	04	08	20
11	11	09	29	14	08	27	17	07	25	19	05	22
12	04	07	32	07	06	30	10	05	28	12	03	25

Tatai Table C (1985–1992)

Month	1985			1986			1987			1988		
	P	S	I	P	S	I	P	S	I	P	S	I
1	04	00	27	07	27	25	10	26	23	13	25	21
2	19	25	29	22	24	27	02	23	25	05	22	23
3	14	25	01	17	24	32	20	23	30	22	21	27
4	06	22	03	09	21	01	12	20	32	14	18	29
5	22	20	06	02	19	04	05	18	02	07	16	32
6	14	17	08	17	16	06	20	15	04	22	13	01
7	07	15	11	10	14	09	13	13	07	15	11	04
8	22	12	13	02	11	11	05	10	09	07	08	06
9	14	09	15	17	08	13	20	07	11	22	05	08
10	07	07	18	10	06	16	13	05	14	15	03	11
11	22	04	20	02	03	18	05	02	16	07	00	13
12	15	02	23	18	01	21	21	00	19	00	26	16

Month	1989			1990			1991			1992		
	P	S	I	P	S	I	P	S	I	P	S	I
1	15	23	18	18	22	16	21	21	14	01	20	12
2	07	20	20	10	19	18	13	18	16	16	17	14
3	02	20	25	05	19	23	08	18	21	10	16	18
4	17	17	27	20	16	25	00	15	23	02	13	20
5	10	15	30	13	14	28	16	13	26	18	11	23
6	02	12	32	05	11	30	08	10	28	10	08	25
7	18	10	02	21	09	00	01	08	31	03	06	28
8	10	07	04	13	06	02	16	05	00	18	03	30
9	02	04	06	05	03	04	08	02	02	10	00	32
10	18	02	09	21	01	07	01	00	05	03	26	02
11	10	27	11	13	26	09	16	25	07	18	23	04
12	03	25	14	06	24	12	09	23	10	11	21	07

Tatai Table C (1993–2000)

Month	1993			1994			1995			1996		
	P	S	I	P	S	I	P	S	I	P	S	I
1	03	18	09	06	17	07	09	16	05	12	15	03
2	18	15	11	21	14	09	01	13	07	04	12	05
3	13	15	16	16	14	14	19	13	12	21	11	09
4	05	12	18	08	11	16	11	10	14	13	08	11
5	21	10	21	01	09	19	04	08	17	06	06	14
6	13	07	23	16	06	21	19	05	19	21	03	16
7	06	05	26	09	04	24	12	03	22	14	01	19
8	21	02	28	01	01	26	04	00	24	06	26	21
9	13	27	30	16	26	28	19	25	26	21	23	23
10	06	25	00	09	24	31	12	23	29	14	21	26
11	21	22	02	01	21	00	04	20	31	06	18	28
12	14	20	05	17	19	03	20	18	01	22	16	31

Month	1997			1998			1999			2000		
	P	S	I	P	S	I	P	S	I	P	S	I
1	14	13	00	17	12	31	20	11	29	00	10	27
2	06	10	02	09	09	00	12	08	31	15	07	29
3	01	10	07	04	09	05	07	08	03	09	06	00
4	16	07	09	19	06	07	22	05	05	01	03	02
5	09	05	12	12	04	10	15	03	08	17	01	05
6	01	02	14	04	01	12	07	00	10	09	26	07
7	17	00	17	20	27	15	00	26	13	02	24	10
8	09	25	19	12	24	17	15	23	15	17	21	12
9	01	22	21	04	21	19	07	20	17	09	18	14
10	17	20	24	20	19	22	00	18	20	02	16	17
11	09	17	26	12	16	24	15	15	22	17	13	19
12	02	15	29	05	14	27	08	13	25	10	11	22

Tatai Table C (2001–2008)

Month	2001			2002			2003			2004		
	P	S	I	P	S	I	P	S	I	P	S	I
1	02	08	24	05	07	22	08	06	20	11	05	18
2	17	05	26	20	04	24	00	03	22	03	02	20
3	12	05	31	15	04	29	18	03	27	20	01	24
4	04	02	00	07	01	31	10	00	29	12	26	26
5	20	00	03	00	27	01	03	26	32	05	24	29
6	12	25	05	15	24	03	18	23	01	20	21	31
7	05	23	08	08	22	06	11	21	04	13	19	01
8	20	20	10	00	19	08	03	18	06	05	16	03
9	12	17	12	15	16	10	18	15	08	20	13	05
10	05	15	15	08	14	13	11	13	11	13	11	08
11	20	12	17	00	11	15	03	10	13	05	08	10
12	13	10	20	16	09	18	19	08	16	21	06	13

Month	2005			2006			2007			2008		
	P	S	I	P	S	I	P	S	I	P	S	I
1	13	03	15	16	02	13	19	01	11	22	00	09
2	05	00	17	08	27	15	11	26	13	14	25	11
3	00	00	22	03	27	20	06	26	18	08	24	15
4	15	25	24	18	24	22	21	23	20	00	21	17
5	08	23	27	11	22	25	14	21	23	16	19	20
6	00	20	29	03	19	27	06	18	25	08	16	22
7	16	18	32	19	17	30	22	16	28	01	14	25
8	08	15	01	11	14	32	14	13	30	16	11	27
9	00	12	03	03	11	01	06	10	32	08	08	29
10	16	10	06	19	09	04	22	08	02	01	06	32
11	08	07	08	11	06	06	14	05	04	16	03	01
12	01	05	11	04	04	09	07	03	07	09	01	04

Tatai Table C (2009–2016)

Month	2009			2010			2011			2012		
	P	S	I	P	S	I	P	S	I	P	S	I
1	01	26	06	04	25	04	07	24	02	10	23	00
2	16	23	08	19	22	06	22	21	04	02	20	02
3	11	23	13	14	22	11	17	21	09	19	19	06
4	03	20	15	06	19	13	09	18	11	11	16	08
5	19	18	18	22	17	16	02	16	14	04	14	11
6	11	15	20	14	14	18	17	13	16	19	11	13
7	04	13	23	07	12	21	10	11	19	12	09	16
8	19	10	25	22	09	23	02	08	21	04	06	18
9	11	07	27	14	06	25	17	05	23	19	03	20
10	04	05	30	07	04	28	10	03	26	12	01	23
11	19	02	32	22	01	30	02	00	28	04	26	25
12	12	00	02	15	27	00	18	26	31	20	24	28

Month	2013			2014			2015			2016		
	P	S	I	P	S	I	P	S	I	P	S	I
1	12	21	30	15	20	28	18	19	26	21	18	24
2	04	18	32	07	17	30	10	16	28	13	15	26
3	22	18	04	02	17	02	05	16	00	07	14	30
4	14	15	06	17	14	04	20	13	02	22	11	32
5	07	13	09	10	12	07	13	11	05	15	09	02
6	22	10	11	02	09	09	05	08	07	07	06	04
7	15	08	14	18	07	12	21	06	10	00	04	07
8	07	05	16	10	04	14	13	03	12	15	01	09
9	22	02	18	02	01	16	05	00	14	07	26	11
10	15	00	21	18	27	19	21	26	17	00	24	14
11	07	25	23	10	24	21	13	23	19	15	21	16
12	00	23	26	03	22	24	06	21	22	08	19	19

Tatai Table C (2017–2024)

Month	2017			2018			2019			2020		
	P	S	I	P	S	I	P	S	I	P	S	I
1	00	16	21	03	15	19	06	14	17	09	13	15
2	15	13	23	18	12	21	21	11	19	01	10	17
3	10	13	28	13	12	26	16	11	24	18	09	21
4	02	10	30	05	09	28	08	08	26	10	06	23
5	18	08	00	21	07	31	01	06	29	03	04	26
6	10	05	02	13	04	00	16	03	31	18	01	28
7	03	03	05	06	02	03	09	01	01	11	27	31
8	18	00	07	21	27	05	01	26	03	03	24	00
9	10	25	09	13	24	07	16	23	05	18	21	02
10	03	23	12	06	22	10	09	21	08	11	19	05
11	18	20	14	21	19	12	01	18	10	03	16	07
12	11	18	17	14	17	15	17	16	13	19	14	10

Month	2021			2022			2023			2024		
	P	S	I	P	S	I	P	S	I	P	S	I
1	11	11	12	14	10	10	17	09	08	20	08	06
2	03	08	14	06	07	12	09	06	10	12	05	08
3	21	08	19	01	07	17	04	06	15	06	04	12
4	13	05	21	16	04	19	19	03	17	21	01	14
5	06	03	24	09	02	22	12	01	20	14	27	17
6	21	00	26	01	27	24	04	26	22	06	24	19
7	14	26	29	17	25	27	20	24	25	22	22	22
8	06	23	31	09	22	29	12	21	27	14	19	24
9	21	20	00	01	19	31	04	18	29	06	16	26
10	14	18	03	17	17	01	20	16	32	22	14	29
11	06	15	05	09	14	03	12	13	01	14	11	31
12	22	13	08	02	12	06	05	11	04	07	09	01

Bibliography

Appel, Walter A. *Biorhythmik*. München: Moderne Verlags Gesellschaft, 1975.

Bochow, Reinhold. "Der Unfall im landwirtschaftlichen Betrieb. Untersuchung über seine Erschening, Ursache und Auswirkung." *Wissenschaftliche Zeitschrift der Humboldt-Universität zu Berlin*. Bd. 4, Nr. 6, pp. 507–39, 1954–55.

Birzele, Karl. *Sonnenaktivität und Biorhythmus des Menschen*. Wien: Franz Deuticke, 1966.

Cold Spring Harbor Symposia on Quantitative Biology. Vol. 25, *Biological Clocks*. New York: Long Island Biological Association, 1960.

Döring, Gerd K. und Schäffers, E. "Über die Tagesrhythmik der Pupillenweite beim Menschen." *Pflügers Archiv für gesamte Physiologie*, Bd. 252, pp. 537–41, 1950.

Douglas E. Neil and Parsons, Stuart O. *Biorhythms—Possible Application to Flight Safety*. A Paper Presented at the International Air Transport Association Twentieth Technical Conference "Safety in Flight Operations." Turkey: November 10–15, 1975.

Dubos, René. *Man Adapting*. New Haven: Yale University Press, 1965.

Frauchger, E. "Rhythmus und Takt in der Lehre vom Leben bei Klages." Verhandlungen der Vierten Konferenz der Internationalen Gesellschaft für Biologische Rhythmus-forschung, Basel: September p. 18–19, 1953.

Früh, Hans R. *Sieg der Lebensrhythmen*. Freiburg: Hermann Bauer Verlag, und Bern; 3 Auflage, Buch-und Offsetdruck Durisch, 1971.

Früh, Hans. *Keine Angust vor der Operation*. Oberhofen: 2 Auflage, Schriftenreihe der Schweiz. Gesellschaft für Periodischelehre und Forschung, 1971.

Ginott, Haim G. *Teacher and Child*. Congruent Communication, 1972.

Gross, Hugo Max. *Biorhythmik*. Freiburg: Hermann Bauer Verlag, 1966.

Heckert, H. "Die Bedeutung der statistischen Darstellungsweise und die Sicherung des Ergebnisses bei der Untersuchung synodisch-lunarer Rhythmen." Verhandlungen der Fünften Konferenz der Internationalen Gesellschaft für Biologische Rhythmusforschung, Stockholm; September pp. 15–17, 1955.

Heinrich, H. W. *Industrial Accident Prevention*. New York: McGraw-Hill, 1931.

Hellpach, Willy. *Geopsyche*. Leipzig; Verlag von Wilhelm Engelmann, 1935.

Hersey, Rex B. "Periodic Emotional Changes in Male Workers." Vol. 7, pp. 459–64, *Personnel Journal*, 1929.

———"Rate of Production and Emotional State." Vol. 10, pp. 355–64, *Personel Journal*, 1932.

———"Emotional Factors in Accidents." Vol. 15, pp. 59–65, *Personnel Journal*, 1936.

Hilliard, Marion. *A Woman Doctor Looks at Love and Life*. New York: Doubleday, 1957.

Kärcher, Adolf, "Biorhythmikdokumentation zur Biorhythmik-Tagung." Leitung von Tatai, Kichinosuke und Kärcher, Adolf. Böblingen: September, 12–15, 1975.

———*Biorhythmik-Wiederentedeckung und Bestätigung der Fliess'schen Periodenlehre*. A Paper Presented at the 7th International Interdisciplinary Cycle Research Symposium. Germany: June 27–July 3, 1976.

Kinugawa, Nobuo, "Accident Analysis in Highschool Physical Education." Sapporo: *Seishutandai-Kiyo*, No. 4, 1973. (In Japanese)

Klages, Ludwig. *Vom Wesen des Rhythmus*. Zürich: 2. Auflage, Verlag Gropengiesser, 1944.

Luthe, Wolfgang (ed.). *Autogenesis Training*. Stuttgart: Georg Thieme Verlag, 1965.

Mason, John W. "Organization of Psychoendocrine Mechanisms." *Psychosomatic Medicine*, Vol. 30, pp. 565–791, 1968.

McDougall, William. *Body and Mind*. London: Methuen Publishers, 1938.

McFarland, Ross A. *Human Factors in Air Transportation*. New York: McGraw-Hill, 1953.

Mears, Ainslie. *Relief without Drugs*. New York: Doubleday, 1967.

Okimura, Yoshiyuki, and Tatai, Kichinosuke. *Biorhythm for Mother and Child*. Osaka: Sankoshobo, 1974. (In Japanese)

Richter, Curt P. "Periodic Phenomena in Man and Animals." In P. R. Michael (ed.), *Endocrinology and Human Behavior*. London: Oxford Press, 1968.

Schwing, Hang. *Über Biorhythmen und deren technische Anwendung*. Zürich: Leemann, 1939.

Selye, Hans. *The Stress of Life*. New York: McGraw-Hill, 1956.

Sollberger, Arne. *Biological Rhythm Research*. Amsterdam: Elsevier Publ., 1965.

Steves, Max. *Biorhythmische Verkehrsunfallverhütung*. Bd. 4, p. 116, Deutsche Polizei, 1965.

Tatai, Kichinosuke (ed.). *Biorhythm Information*. Tokyo: Japan Biorhythm Laboratory, 1968–73. (In Japanese)

Tatai, Kichinosuke. *What is Biorhythm*. Tokyo: Kodansha, 1973. (In Japanese)

————*Studies on the Reduction of Automobile Accidents in Applying the Theory of Biorhythmics by Fliess*. A Paper Presented at the 7th International Interdisciplinary Cycle Research Symposium. Germany: June 27–July 3, 1976.

Tope, Otto. *Biorhythmische Einflüsse und ihre Auswirkung in Führparkbetrieben*. Bd. 9, Hannover: Städtehygiene, 1956.

Wernli, Hans J. *Biorhythm*. New York: Crown Publishers, 1961.

Wolf, William (ed.) "Rhythmic Functions in the Living System." *Annals of the New York Academy of Sciences*, Vol. 98, Art. 4, pp. 753–1326, 1962.

Wolff, Harold G. *Stress and Disease*. 2. ed., Springfield: C. C. Thomas, 1968.

Index

Hellbrügge, Theodor, 43
Hemingway, Ernest, 94, 95
Heraclitus, 39
Hersey, Lexford, 17
high-key phase, 60
Hilliard, Marion, 38
Hino, Ashihei, 94
Hippocrates, 19
homeokinesis, 28
homeostasis, 29
Horie, Shigeo, 84
hormone, 14, 15, 17, 28, 29, 35, 36, 39
human relation, 114
Husserl, Edmund, 21
Hypnosis, 34

Ikemi, Torijiro, 30, 32
instruction to children, 120
intellectual cycle, 16
International Interdisciplinary Cycle
  Research Symposium, 101

Jacobson, Edmund, 35, 36
Japan Biorhythm Laboratory, 49, 53,
  55, 59, 68, 73, 74, 84, 88, 100
Journal of Interdisciplinary Cycle Research,
  20
Judt, Alffred, 17, 48
Judt-Früh Simplified Calculation Table,
  55
Judt-Früh system, 49
Judt table, 52
Juro, Evan, 19

Kaiser, I. H., 44
Kämmerle, K., 97
Kärcher, Adolf, 101, 106, 108, 121
Kawabata, Yasunari, 96
Kawai, Minoru, 108
Klages, Ludwig, 21, 38, 39
Komarov (cosmonaut), 80, 81
Krayenbuhl, H., 102
Kubo, Masao, 108
Kurosawa, Akira, 94, 95

Latané, Bibb, 35
Law of Initial Value (LIV), 65
law of moderation, 112
life cycle, 11
Life Destructive Behavior Test, 98, 99
life rhythm, 11, 39
low-key phase, 60, 65, 66
Luthe, Wolfgang, 30, 31

manegerial sickness, 15
Mansfield, Jayne, 104
Mantle, Mickey, 38
Margaret (Princess), 105
Mason, W., 35
Mathieu, Mireille, 126
McFarland, Ross A., 79, 83, 92
McGregor, Douglas, 114
Meares, Ainslie, 32
menstrual cycle, 22, 23, 25, 28
Meyfarth, Ulrike, 110
mini-Zen, 36, 37
Mishima Yukio, 95, 96
Monteran, Henri, 94, 95
monthly cycle in common diseases, 24
moon-related monthly cycle, 23
motivation, 31, 32, 125
Munich Olympics, 107, 110

Nachtarbeiterkrankheit, 14
Naegle's law, 27, 105
Nagashima, Shigeo, 108
negative phase, 73, 74
Neil, Dougles E., 121
neobiorhythm, 125
neo-Fliessian, 124
nervous system, 13, 66
Niedom, Joseph, 125
night-work sickness, 14
Nixon, Richard, 20
noradrenalin, 35, 39, 123, 129, 140
Nordwig, Wolfgang, 110

Oba, Masao, 87, 88
Okimura, Yoshiyuki, 118, 119, 121, 123
Oparin, Aleksandr Ivanovich, 11
operation, 100, 101
Osanai, Masao, 84, 88, 89

physical cycle, 16
Pierach, Alexander, 14
Pocket Biorhythm Calendar, 70
Portmann, Adolf, 27
positive phase, 73, 74
Pozien, P., 31, 32
predicting birth, 105
PSI cycle, 25
PSI theory, 15, 16, 19, 21, 38, 139

Quételet, Adolphe, 46, 48

Rautenstrauch, 106
reading efficiency, 14
reduction of air accidents, 80
reduction of traffic accidents, 39, 51, 83
relaxation, 35–37

Physical Cycle (twenty-three days) Especially important for sportsmen, people engaged in strenuous activity, and ill persons.	Positive phase	Abundant stamina	Good time for surgical operations and for body-strengthening training, sports contests, travel, or work involving physical strength.
	Caution day	Body conditions unstable	A time when heart attacks, colds, headaches, diarrhea, allergies, and hangovers are likely to occur and when the symptoms of sicknesses can grow worse or accidents can take place.
	Negative phase	Inadequate stamina	A time for ordinary activity and plenty of rest. Control expenditures of energy and avoid overwork.
Sensitivity Cycle (twenty-eight days) Especially important for businessmen, professional sportsmen, and artists.	Positive phase	Abundant vigor	Good time for participating in competitions, taking examinations, holding lectures, performing in public, having dates, proposing to one's sweetheart, and engaging in teamwork.
	Caution day	Emotions unstable	A time when one may either make slips of the tongue or talk too much and get into fights or accidents. Heart attacks, apoplexy, and worsening of illness symptoms are likely to occur at such times.
	Negative phase	Inadequate vigor	Concentrate on ordinary work and the tidying up of odds and ends of office work. Be cautious in relations with other people.
Intellectual Cycle (thirty-three days) Especially important to students, scholars, managerial workers, and politicians.	Positive phase	Full intellectual powers	A good time to undertake new work, make plans, devise experiments, discuss and undertake political strategies, or initiate studies in new fields.
	Caution day	Intellectual powers unstable	Powers of memory and intuition decrease. One becomes forgetful and tends to make blunders and be absentminded.
	Negative phase	Intellectual powers in a slump	One should concentrate on such work as adjusting and collecting data and should not over tax one's mind.